Clinical Research in
Gastroenterology 1

Clinical Research in Gastroenterology 1

edited by

S. Matern

Chairman of the Third Department of Internal Medicine
Medical Faculty of Aachen University of Technology
Aachen, West Germany

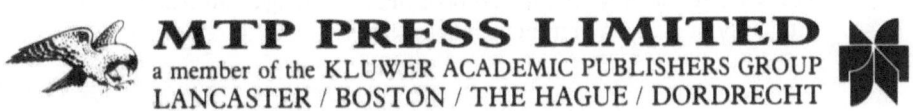

MTP PRESS LIMITED
a member of the KLUWER ACADEMIC PUBLISHERS GROUP
LANCASTER / BOSTON / THE HAGUE / DORDRECHT

Published in the UK and Europe by
MTP Press Limited
Falcon House
Lancaster, England

British Library Cataloguing in Publication Data
Clinical research in gastroenterology 1.
  1. Gastrointestinal system—Diseases
  I. Matern, S.
  616.3′3   RC801

  ISBN-13: 978-94-010-7937-2   e-ISBN-13: 978-94-009-3203-6
  DOI: 10.1007/978-94-009-3203-6
Published in the USA by
MTP Press
A division of Kluwer Academic Publishers
101 Philip Drive
Norwell, MA 02061, USA

Library of Congress Cataloging in Publication Data
Clinical research in gastroenterology 1.
  Includes bibliographies and index.
  1. Gastrointestinal system—Diseases.
I. Matern, S. [DNLM: 1. Gastrointestinal
Diseases. WI 100 C641]
RC801.C57 1987   616.3   87–3238

Contents

List of Authors

H. E. Blum
Department of Medicine
University of Freiburg
Hugstetter Strasse 55
D-7800 Freiburg
West Germany

M. Classen
II Medizinische Klinik und
  Poliklinik der Technischen
  Universität München
Klinikum rechts der Isar
Ismaninger Strasse 22
D-8000 München 80
West Germany

H. Dancygier
II Medizinische Klinik und
  Poliklinik der Technischen
  Universität München
Klinikum rechts der Isar
Ismaninger Strasse 22
D-8000 München 80
West Germany

W. Gerok
Department of Medicine
University of Freiburg
Hugstetter Strasse 55
D-7800 Freiburg
West Germany

G. Lux
I Medizinische Klinik
Gotenstrasse 1
D-5650 Solingen
West Germany

G. A. Mannes
II Medizinische Klinik Gross-
  hadern
Universität München
Marchioninistrasse 15
D-8000 München 70
West Germany

S. Matern
Internal Medicine III
RWTH Aachen
Pauwelstrasse
D-5100 Aachen
West Germany

G. Paumgartner
II Medizinische Klinik Gross-
  hadern
Universität München
D-8000 München 70
Marchioninistrasse 15
West Germany

F. Stellaard
UU-Fiehenhuis
Laboratorium Kindergenees-
  kunde
De Boeldaan 1117
1007 MB Amsterdam
The Netherlands

H. Wietholtz
Internal Medicine III
RWTH Aachen
Pauwelstrasse
D-5100 Aachen
West Germany

Preface

The last decade has seen tremendous developments in many fields of gastroenterology and hepatology. The aim of this series is to highlight some of these topics that deserve particular interest.

Research in the field of viral hepatitis has been very intense and successful in recent years. The hepatitis B virus is one of the best explored at the current level of virology. Not only the nucleotid sequence of the viral DNA can be decoded, but also the amino acid compounds of its genetic products are known today. Since the techniques of molecular biology have increasingly found access to clinical laboratory use, hepatitis B virus infection can serve as an example for the importance of molecular biology in clinical hepatology.

Another example for the interdependence of basic science and clinical medicine represents the research on bile acid metabolism. The investigation of bile acids has revealed new diagnostic approaches to hepatic and intestinal disorders. Commercial kits for the routine measurement of serum bile acids in clinical laboratories by enzymatic or radioimmunologic techniques are now available. The diagnostic value of these measurements in gastroenterology and hepatology shall be defined. Another aspect of bile acid research leads to new perspectives in the treatment of gallstone disease. The dissolution of cholesterol gallstones by chenodeoxycholic acid (therapy) may be quoted as the best example for the development of new pharmacotherapeutic principles derived from basic bile acid research. At present many therapeutic agents are used to dissolve gallstones not only in the gallbladder but also in the biliary tract. Therefore recent advances on formation and dissolution of biliary calculi will be discussed.

Another field of rapid development in recent years has been that of operative endoscopy and endoscopic ultrasound. Endoscopic laser therapy has been used in the treatment of gastrointestinal haemorrhage. It is well established in the therapy of bleeding from peptic ulcers and might be of use in angiomatous lesions as well. Finally laser therapy finds more and more clinical application in palliation of gastrointestinal neoplasia and malignancies. In only five years the concept of laser treatment has advanced from a pure research idea to routine use in the management of gastrointestinal conditions. For this reason its place in clinical gastroenterology is indicated. In spite of recent progress in standard diagnostic imaging procedures, the combination of a gastroscope with an ultrasonic probe seems to open new perspectives for the examination of the oesophagus, the stomach, the duodenum and their neighbouring organs. Endoscopic ultrasound could become an important complementary diagnostic method in disorders confined to the gastrointestinal wall, the pancreas and the common bile duct, with particular sensitivity to the papilla of Vater. Therefore the value of this new technique will be reviewed.

Finally I would like to thank those who have participated in this volume for their excellent contributions on their individual fields of expertise. I am indebted to Mrs. Valerie Baker and Dr. Peter Clarke from MTP Press without whose assistance and understanding the organisation of this book would not have been possible.

Siegfried Matern

1

Clinical Significance of Molecular Studies of Hepatitis B Virus Infection

H. E. Blum and W. Gerok

INTRODUCTION

Infection with the hepatitis B virus (HBV) is endemic throughout much of the world with an estimated 200 million persistently infected people[1-5]. HBV infects only humans and certain non-human primates, and belongs to a group of *hepa*totropic *DNA* (hepadna) viruses that includes the hepatitis virus of the woodchuck[6], the Beechey ground squirrel[7], and the Pekin duck[8]. In humans, HBV infection is associated with a wide spectrum of clinical presentations, ranging from the clinically inapparent 'healthy' carrier state, to acute and fulminant hepatitis, to various forms of chronic liver disease and to liver cirrhosis. Further, HBV infection is clearly involved in the development of hepatocellular carcinoma (HCC), worldwide a leading cause of death from cancer[9-25].

Important advances have been made during the past few years in the study of the biology of HBV and the virus/host cell interaction at the molecular level. The HBV genome has been cloned by recombinant DNA technologies and its detailed structure, including the complete nucleotide sequence, has been determined. The genetic organization of the genome has been established and viral genes have been expressed *in vitro* in various cell culture systems. Using cloned HBV DNA, viral

1

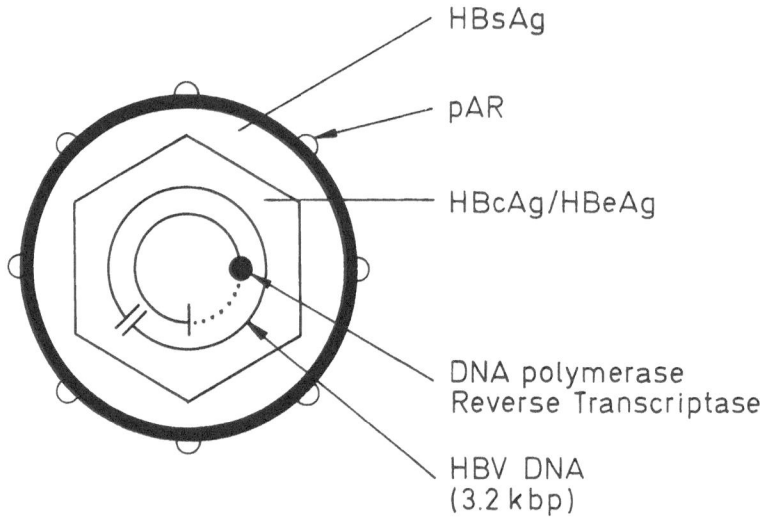

Fig. 1.1 Structure of hepatitis B virus (HBsAg, hepatitis B surface antigen; pAR, polyalbumin receptor; HBcAg, hepatitis B core antigen; HBeAg, hepatitis B e antigen; kbp, kilobase pairs)

nucleic acids have been identified and characterized in serum and liver of individuals infected by HBV using molecular hybridization techniques. These techniques have revealed two new and exciting aspects of the biology of HBV: the existence of HBV DNA in serum and liver of HBsAg-negative patients with liver disease (non-A, non-B hepatitis) and the presence of HBV DNA in non-hepatocytes. We will briefly review the structure, genetic organization and mode of replication of the HBV. Then we will describe recent developments in the laboratory diagnosis of HBV infection by molecular hybridization analyses and their significance for a clinical understanding of the pathogenetic mechanisms leading to HBV-induced liver diseases, including HCC.

STRUCTURE OF HEPATITIS B VIRUS

The hepatitis B virion ('Dane particle') has a diameter of approximately 42 nm[26]. It consists of an electron-dense internal core structure (nucleocapsid) with a diameter of 28 nm and an envelope of about 7 nm thickness (Fig. 1.1). The envelope of the virion carries the hepatitis B surface antigen (HBsAg) which shares antigenic determinants with the incomplete viral particles (22 nm spherical and filamentous empty envelope forms)[27]. Three main serotypes of HBsAg (adw, adr, ayw) are commonly observed with a distinct worldwide distribution[28]. Electrophoretic analysis of HBsAg revealed three proteins called the major, the middle and the large protein[29,30]. These proteins occur in glycosylated/non-glycosylated forms and are encoded by the S gene, the pre-S2/S genes and the pre-S1/pre-S2/S genes, respectively (see below). In addition, the envelope carries a receptor for polymerized human serum albumin[29,31] which is believed to mediate the attachment of HBV to hepatocytes[5].

The nucleocapsid contains the hepatitis B core antigen (HBcAg) and its cryptic antigenic determinant hepatitis B e antigen (HBeAg[32,33]), the viral DNA with a protein covalently attached to the 5'-end of the minus-strand[34], a DNA polymerase/reverse transcriptase[35,36], and a protein kinase[37].

STRUCTURE OF HEPATITIS B VIRUS GENOME

The HBV genome is a small circular DNA molecule of about 3.2 kilobase pairs length[38] (Fig. 1.2). The DNA is only partially double-stranded with a single-stranded region that varies in length between 15 and 60% of the viral genome in different molecules[39-41], displaying a preferred minimum length of 650–700 nucleotides[42]. The complete minus-strand is of constant length of about 3200 nucleotides and has a nick with a protein covalently attached to its 5'-end[34], preventing phosphorylation of the DNA by polynucleotide kinase. The 5'-end of the incomplete plus-strand is about 200–300 nucleotides downstream from the 5'-end of the minus-strand, thus creating a cohesive overlap that maintains the circular structure of virion DNA[39,43-45]. DNAs of this size and structure, including the single-stranded region and a DNA polymerase that functions to fill in the gap by elongation from the 3'-end of the incomplete plus-strand[35,36,39-41] have been found so far only in HBV and the other hepadna viruses of woodchuck[6], ground squirrel[7] and Pekin duck[8].

The DNAs of all four hepadna viruses have been cloned in bacteria[46] and the complete nucleotide sequences of HBV[47-50], woodchuck[51,52] and Pekin duck[53,54] DNAs have been established.

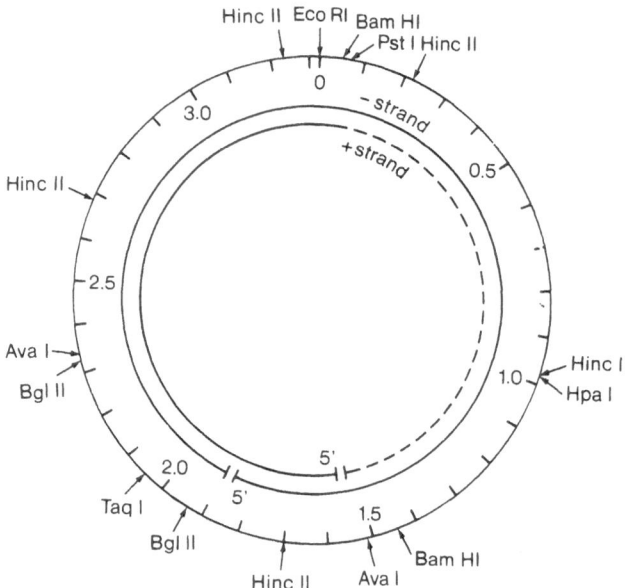

Fig. 1.2 Physical structure and restriction enzyme cleavage sites of the HBV genome (HBsAg subtype adw2[45])

GENETIC ORGANIZATION OF HEPATITIS B VIRUS GENOME

The minus-strand of virion DNA contains four open reading frames based on the three reading phases of the nucleotide sequence and the position of AUG start and TAA, TGA, or TAG stop codons. A comparison of the nucleotide sequence of the reading frames with the available information on the gene products HBsAg and HBcAg (molecular weight, amino acid composition and sequence) allowed the identification and localization of these viral genes in the viral genome (Fig. 1.3). These coding regions include the region that codes for the three proteins of HBsAg, including the receptor for polymerized human serum albumin (gene S and a contiguous region upstream termed pre-S gene), the region that codes for HBcAg (gene C) and the regions coding for DNA polymerase (gene P) and the X protein (gene X). Through extensive overlapping of gene P with genes pre S/S, X and C (Fig. 1.3) the small HBV genome can code for all known proteins: HBsAg (major, middle and large protein[29,30], HBxAg,

4

HBcAg/HBeAg and DNA polymerase/reverse transcriptase/RNA ase H.

REPLICATION OF HEPATITIS B VIRUS GENOME

Based on work with the Pekin duck hepatitis virus[55,56] replication of HBV is strikingly different from all other animal DNA viruses and involves the reverse transcription of an RNA intermediate by a virus-encoded reverse transcriptase. This replication strategy is characteristic for the (RNA-containing) retroviruses, many of which are tumour viruses[57].

Upon internalization into host cells the infecting, partially single-stranded viral genome is made double-stranded, adopts a superhelical conformation and serves as template for the transcription of its minus-strand into viral RNA by a cellular RNA polymerase. These viral RNA molecules serve either as messenger RNA (mRNA) or as template ('pregenome') for the reverse transcription into minus-strand DNA. These reverse-transcribed minus-strand DNA species, synthesized by HBV reverse transcriptase, are then made partially double-stranded by the viral DNA polymerase to give mature virion DNA[56,59]. Viral DNA replication is therefore asymmetric with separate pathways for minus- and plus-strand DNA syntheses and involves the reverse transcription of an RNA intermediate[5,56,59]. In addition to the Pekin duck hepatitis virus[55,56], this mechanism has now been demonstrated to be operative also in ground squirrel hepatitis virus[58,59] and the human/chimpanzee HBV[60-63], indicating that this mode of replication is central to the life cycle of all hepadna viruses.

MOLECULAR HYBRIDIZATION ANALYSES

Molecular hybridization techniques, using cloned HBV DNA as a probe, allow quantitative and qualitative analyses related to the detection, characterization and localization of viral nucleic acid sequences in serum, cells or tissues. The principle of all hybridization analyses is the formation of a hybrid between nucleic acids from serum, cells or tissues and radiolabelled cloned HBV DNA through complementary base pairing. The radiolabelled hybrid molecules can then be detected by autoradiography.

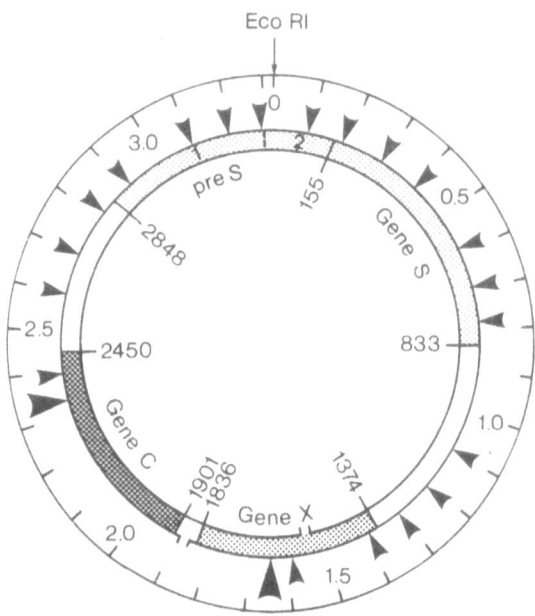

Fig. 1.3 Genetic organization of HBV genome and localization of HBV genes pre-S1, pre-S2, S, X, C and P (DNA polymerase/reverse transcriptase, arrows)

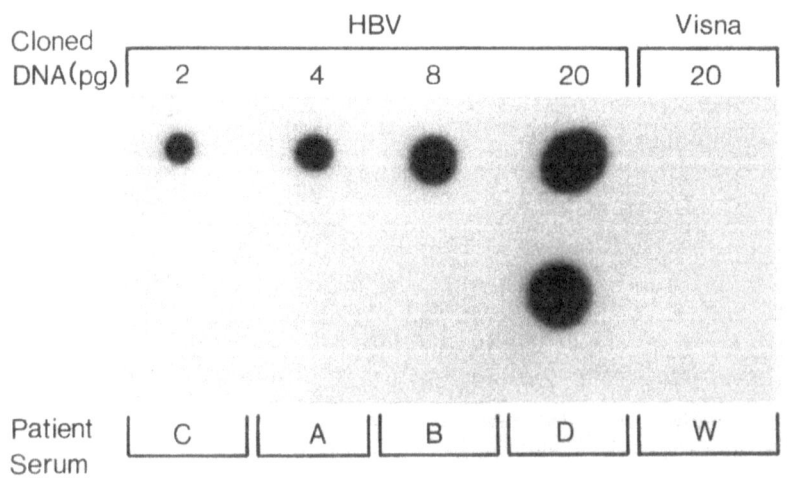

Fig. 1.4 Dot blot hybridization analysis of cloned HBV DNA, Visna cDNA and HBsAg-positive patient sera

Table 1.1 Hybridization techniques: detection and characterization of HBV
DNA/RNA by dot blot, transfer blot and *in situ* hybridization

	Dot blot	Transfer blot (Southern/Northern)	In situ hybridization
DNA	+	+	+
RNA	+	+	+
Quantitation	+	+	+
Characterization:			
RNA size classes	−	+	−
DNA size classes	−	+	−
DNA conformation	−	+	−
DNA integration	−	+	−
Restriction analysis	−	+	−
Replicative forms			
(ssDNA)	+	+	+
Single cell analysis	−	−	+
Tissue pattern of viral			
DNA/RNA transcripts	−	−	+
Detection of rare/focal			
nucleic acid sequences	−	−	+
Combination of			
DNA/RNA			
hybridization with			
immunohistochemistry	−	−	+

These analyses offer a new insight into the biology of HBV in acute
and chronic liver disease, as well as into the oncogenic potential of
HBV as a cause of hepatocellular carcinoma. Three distinct types of
hybridization assays are used, each of which has its particular power
(Table 1.1): dot blot hybridization, transfer blot hybridization and *in
situ* hybridization.

Dot blot hybridization

The principle of this technique is the immobilization of nucleic acids
(DNA/RNA) from serum, cells or tisssues on a membrane, followed
by hybridization with radiolabelled cloned HBV DNA. Annealing of
viral DNA/RNA to the HBV-specific probe results in radiolabelled
hybrid molecules which can be detected by autoradiography and

quantitated by densitometry or liquid scintillation counting, relative to standards of known amounts of cloned viral DNA (Fig. 1.4).

The dot blot hybridization assay is specific for the detection of HBV DNA since an unrelated radiolabelled probe (e.g. pBR 322 DNA) or DNA from an unrelated virus (e.g. Visna cDNA) do not result in a detectable hybrid formation as illustrated in Fig. 1.4.

This assay is easy to perform and readily identifies HBV DNA in the serum from an HBV carrier, serologically positive for HBsAg, HBeAg and anti-HBc (patient serum D, Fig. 1.4). This result unequivocally demonstrates active viral replication in this patient's liver and is indicative for a high risk of transmitting HBV infection to others, especially to recipients of blood or blood products and to close personal contacts. In contrast, three patients serologically positive for HBsAg, anti-HBe and anti-HBc (patient sera C, A, B and W, Fig. 1.4) are negative for serum HBV DNA.

Transfer blot hybridization

The principle of this technique is the separation of DNA or RNA molecules according to size by electrophoresis through agarose, followed by transfer to a nucleic acid binding membrane under conditions preserving the relative positions of the DNA or RNA species in the gel. The immobilized DNA or RNA molecules are then hybridized with a radiolabelled HBV DNA probe. The presence and position of the nucleic acid species complementary to the probe is then detected by autoradiography. This technique was first described in 1975 for the analysis of DNA molecules[64] and popularly termed Southern blot analysis. In keeping with this terminology, the transfer blots for the characterization of RNA molecules were then termed Northern blots.

Southern blot analyses of DNA extracted from liver tissues have been extensively used in characterization of the state of HBV DNA in various forms of liver disease. These studies have demonstrated that HBV DNA in hepatocytes can exist in free, extrachromosomal, actively replicating forms as well as covalently integrated into the cellular genome.

The hybridization pattern of DNA extracted from the liver of a patient with active viral replication is characterized by the presence of DNA molecules of full length (3.2 kilobase pairs) and large amounts

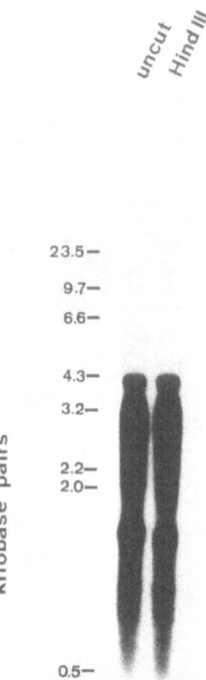

Fig. 1.5 Southern blot hybridization analysis of DNA extracted from the liver of a patient with HBeAg-positive chronic active hepatitis. Digestion with restriction endonucleases indicated on top

of smaller, nascent nucleic acids (Fig. 1.5). These species were shown to be predominantly single-stranded and of minus-strand polarity, demonstrating the asymmetric replication of the HBV genome (see above). By contrast, in hepatocellular carcinoma HBV DNA is predominantly integrated into the cellular genome. These integrated viral nucleic acid sequences are detectable only after digestion of cellular DNA by restriction endonuclease(s) (Fig. 1.6): as a result of the flanking chromosomal sequences the viral DNA species can have apparent lengths of more than 3.2 kilobase pairs, the unit-length of the free viral genome (see above).

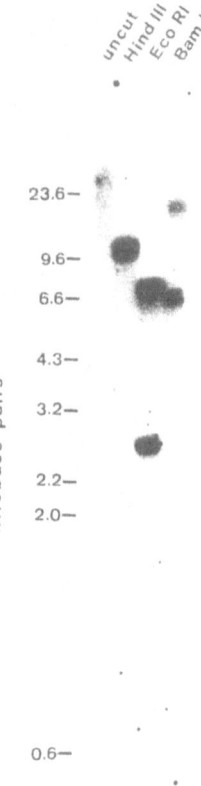

Fig. 1.6 Southern blot hybridization analysis of DNA extracted from a human hepatocellular carcinoma. Digestion with restriction endonucleases indicated on top

In situ hybridization

The principle of this technique is the annealing of single-stranded nucleic acid molecules in tissues, cells or cellular preparations (e.g. chromosomes) to a single-stranded, radiolabelled probe to form a hybrid molecule that can be detected by autoradiography. Because of the combination of molecular hybridization and cytological pro-

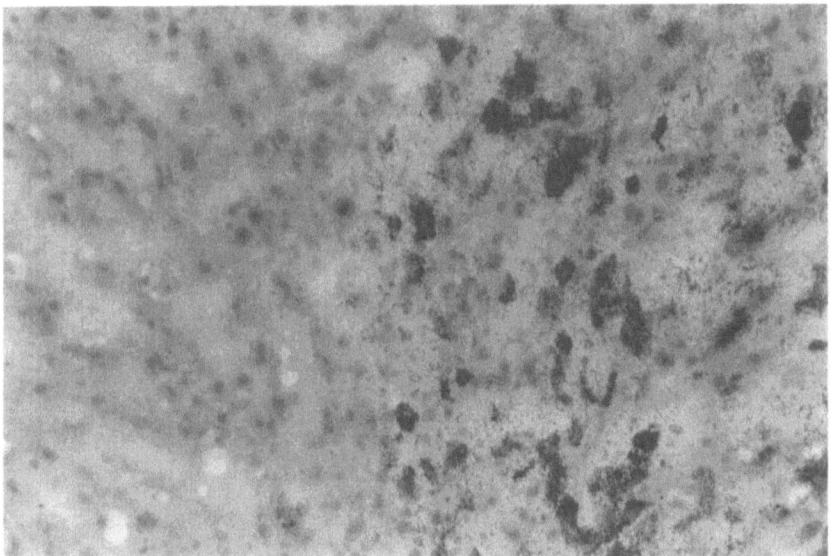

Fig. 1.7 *In situ* hybridization analysis of the liver from a patient with HBeAg-positive chronic active hepatitis.

cedures it is possible to localize genes on chromosomes, to follow their expression in cells and to detect and quantitate viral genes in infected cells.

By this technique HBV DNA is readily detected in infected hepatocytes and shows a highly focal tissue distribution with infected cells next to uninfected cells (Fig. 1.7). Patients with active viral replication display predominantly cytoplasmic hybridization patterns. These cytoplasmic viral nucleic acid species were shown to be mostly single-stranded and of minus-strand polarity, and demonstrate at the cellular level the asymmetric replication of HBV DNA[60].

CLINICAL SIGNIFICANCE OF MOLECULAR HYBRIDIZATION ANALYSES

Dot blot hybridization

The dot blot hybridization assays are specific for the detection of HBV DNA in serum, and viral nucleic acids from cells or tissues. This technique is easy to perform and allows the simultaneous analysis of a virtually unlimited number of samples. If positive, dot blot hybridization unequivocally identifies individuals with high levels of infectious virus in serum, reflecting active viral replication in their liver.

However, due to the relative insensitivity of the dot blot hybridization technique (limit of detection about 0.05 pg HBV DNA, equivalent to 15 000 virus particles), negative results do not exclude the presence of infectious virus in serum or active viral replication in the liver. On the other hand, several studies have now established that dot blot analyses are more sensitive for the detection of HBV in the serum than radioimmunoassay for HBeAg and tests for DNA polymerase activity[65–73,106]. Additionally, HBV DNA has been detected by dot blot analyses in some HBsAg-negative sera with and without antibodies to viral antigens[69,74–76,106]. By contrast, no HBV DNA was detected in sera from patients with acute hepatitis serologically negative for HBsAg and positive for anti-HBc and anti-HBs or with acute hepatitis serologically negative for all viral markers (non-A, non-B hepatitis[71]). Nevertheless, these findings provide remarkable evidence that some HBsAg-positive/HBeAg-negative patients, and HBsAg-negative individuals with or without antibodies to HBV antigens (non-A, non-B hepatitis) may have active HBV replication in their livers and have to be considered potentially infectious. Dot blot hybridization thus provides a sensitive and direct means of detecting HBV in serum. These results redefine the classical serological patterns of HBV infection and are epidemiologically very important in identifying individuals with HBV DNA in serum, irrespective of their HBsAg, HBeAg or anti-HBe status (Tables 1.2 and 1.3), indicating a high risk of transmitting HBV infection to recipients of blood or blood products and to close personal contacts.

Dot blot hybridization can also be applied for the detection of viral DNA or RNA extracted from cells, tissues or subcellular fractions. As an analysis preliminary to a more detailed characterization of viral nucleic acid sequences by transfer blots, dot blot hybridization allows the specific demonstration of HBV DNA or RNA and the calculation of the average number of viral copies per ml serum or per cell.

Transfer blot hybridization

The presence and state of viral DNA/RNA in liver tissues have been studied in detail by transfer blot hybridizations. Southern blot analyses

Table 1.2 HBV DNA in serum from HBsAg-positive patients with chronic hepatitis (A[69] and B[67])

	HBsAg	HBeAg	Anti-HBe	HBV DNA positive
Hepatitis A				
	+	+	−	96% (52/54)
	+	−	+	63% (14/22)
	+	−	−	66% (2/3)
Hepatitis B				
	+	+	−	100% (10/10)
	+	−	+	54% (13/24)

Table 1.3 HBV DNA in serum from HBsAg-negative patients with chronic hepatitis[76]

HBsAg	Anti-HBc	Anti-HBs	HBV DNA positive
−	+	+	3.8% (4/105)
−	+	−	5.7% (6/105)
		Total	9.5% (10/105)

of DNA extracted from liver tissue have been extensively used in characterization of the state of HBV DNA in various forms of liver disease. These studies have demonstrated that HBV DNA in hepatocytes can exist in free, extrachromosomal forms as well as integrated into the cellular genome.

Free viral DNA has been generally found in the liver of HBeAg-positive patients[12,60,62,63,70] while integrated forms are predominantly associated with HBe-negative chronic liver disease and HCC[10,12,17,21–25,78].

However, not all HCCs in patients with past or present HBV infection contain viral DNA integrated into the cellular genome[79,80].

On the other hand, HBV DNA has been demonstrated in the liver of some patients with HBsAg-negative liver disease with or without

Table 1.4   HBV DNA in non-hepatocytes

Cells/tissues	Reference
Bile duct epithelium, endothelial and smooth muscle cells of the liver	101
Spleen	102
Lymphoblastoid cells	83–85
Peripheral blood mononuclear cells	86–89, 93, 94
Pancreas, kidney, skin	90
Kaposi's sarcoma	95

antibodies to HBV antigens[10,12,74–76,81], but not in others[82]. These findings suggest that at least in some cases of serologically defined non-A, non-B hepatitis, the chronic liver disease may in fact be caused by HBV or HBV-related agents.

Southern blot analyses of liver DNA thus provide a powerful method for the detection and characterization of viral DNA species in various forms of HBV-related liver disease, including HCC, and permit the study of the interaction of the virus with the host cell at the molecular level. Further, HBV DNA has been demonstrated in cells other than hepatocytes (Table 1.4): in lymphoblastoid cells[83–85], peripheral blood mononuclear cells[86–89,93,94], pancreas, kidney and skin[90] of HBV-infected individuals. Also, in the chimpanzee and woodchuck models of hepatitis B, viral DNA was detected in peripheral blood lymphocytes[91]. HBV DNA has been further detected in saliva, urine and seminal fluid of carriers of HBeAg[92]. Finally, HBV DNA sequences were found in lymphoid cells[93] and in peripheral blood mononuclear cells[94] of patients with acquired immune deficiency syndrome (AIDS) and AIDS-related complex, and in Kaposi's sarcoma[95]. All these findings indicate that the host cell range for HBV is more extensive than has been appreciated previously. The biological significance and pathological potential of the presence of HBV DNA in non-hepatocytes, however, remain to be defined.

In situ hybridization

At the tissue and single cell level viral nucleic acid sequences can be detected by *in situ* hybridization. *In situ* hybridization has been applied

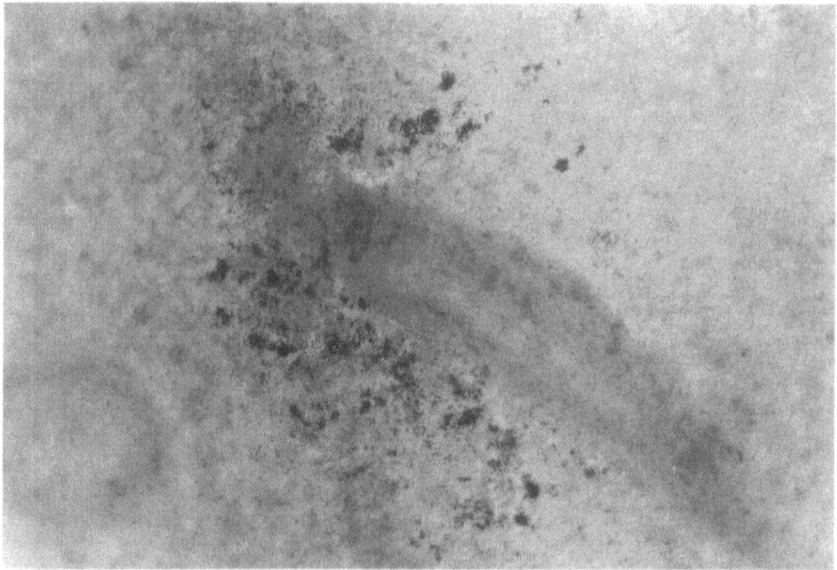

Fig. 1.8 *In situ* hybridization analysis of the spleen from a patient with HBeAg-positive chronic active hepatitis

for the study of HBV-related liver disease in tissues and HBV DNA containing cell lines[96-105]. The technique has proven to be specific for detection of HBV DNA or RNA since hybridization with an unrelated probe (e.g. pBR 322 DNA) or to uninfected human liver results in a negative hybridization signal. This assay is highly sensitive and detects as little as about 5 HBV genome equivalents per cell, as determined by comparative hybridization analyses of human hepatoma cells (PLC/PRF/5; Alexander cells) which contain about four copies of HBV DNA integrated into the cellular genome[101].

Due to the high sensitivity of the *in situ* hybridization assay and visualization of the infected cells, HBV DNA could be demonstrated not only in hepatocytes but also in the bile duct epithelium, in endothelial cells and smooth muscle cells of blood vessel walls in HBV-infected liver as well as in the spleen[101,102] (Fig. 1.8). This assay has identified new target cells for HBV infection, extending the known host cell range for HBV. These findings are of particular significance for the understanding of the biology of HBV and are consistent with several recent reports demonstrating HBV in various non-hepatocytes (Table 1.4).

The *in situ* hybridization assay thus provides a specific and sensitive tool for the localization and quantitation of viral nucleic acids at the single cell level and for the identification of individuals with active replication of HBV DNA hitherto not possible with other nucleic acid hybridization analyses. This assay is particularly useful since it requires only a fraction of a liver needle biopsy obtained routinely for diagnostic purposes, and should permit following the natural course of HBV infection and selecting and monitoring patients undergoing antiviral therapies.

SUMMARY AND PERSPECTIVES

The HBV genome consists of a small circular, partially double-stranded DNA molecule of about 3200 nucleotides length. The physical structure and localization of the major genes of HBV have been identified and the complete nucleotide sequence of the HBV genome has been established. The viral genome replicates asymmetrically with separate pathways for the minus- and plus-strand synthesis and involves the reverse transcription of an RNA intermediate as a central feature of its replication strategy, characteristic for the (RNA-containing) retroviruses, many of which are tumour viruses[57].

HBV infection in humans is associated with a wide spectrum of clinical presentations, ranging from the clinically inapparent, 'healthy' carrier state, to acute/fulminant hepatitis, various forms of chronic hepatitis and liver cirrhosis to hepatocellular carcinoma. Currently, the specific laboratory diagnosis of HBV infection is based on the serological detection of HBsAg, HBeAg/anti-HBe, anti-HBc and anti-HBs. Three newly developed molecular hybridization techniques have permitted: (1) the direct identification of HBV DNA in serum by dot blot analysis; (2) the characterization of viral nucleic acid sequences with respect to their interaction with the host cells (free, extra-chromosomal *vs.* integrated viral DNA) by Southern blots; and (3) the localization and quantitation of viral nucleic acid sequences at the single cell level by *in situ* hybridization, combined with the immunohistochemical visualization of viral antigens[103]. These analyses permit a comprehensive assessment of the biology of HBV at the genetic (DNA), transcriptional (RNA) and translational (anti-gens/proteins) levels.

The clinical significance of the molecular analyses of HBV infection lies:

1. in the detection of active viral replication by demonstration and characterization of HBV nucleic acids in serum and/or liver of patients with HBV infection;
2. in the estimation of the infectivity of patients with HBV infection and their potential risk to others[106];
3. in the possibility of following the natural course of HBV infection[71-73,107-109] and to assess the effectiveness of antiviral or immunosuppressive therapy[110-118];
4. in the detection of integrated HBV DNA in hepatocellular carcinoma from patients serologically positive or negative for HBV markers, suggesting a pathogenetic role of HBV in the mechanisms leading to the malignant transformation of hepatocytes;
5. in the demonstration of HBV as an aetiologic agent in serum and/or liver from patients with HBsAg-negative liver disease, some of whom are negative for all markers of HBV infection (non-A, non-B hepatitis);
6. in the detection of viral nucleic acids in non-hepatocytes from patients with or without serological evidence of past or present HBV infection.

With increasing knowledge of the structural and biological characteristics of HBV we shall gain more insight into the pathogenetic mechanisms leading to acute and fulminant liver cell injury, to viral persistence and chronic liver disease, including hepatocellular carcinoma. While HBV replication does not seem to be directly cytopathic, several lines of evidence suggest that immune mechanisms are involved in the pathogenesis of HBV-associated liver cell injury[119-123].

References

1. Robinson, W. S. (1977). The genome of hepatitis B virus. *Ann. Rev. Microbiol.*, **31**, 357–77
2. McCollum, R. W. and Zuckerman, A. J. (1981). Viral hepatitis: Report on a WHO informal consultation. *J. Med. Virol.*, **8**, 1–29

3. Tiollais, P., Charnay, P. and Vyas, G. N. (1981). Biology of hepatitis B virus. *Science.*, **213**, 406–11

4. Vyas, G. N. and Blum, H. E. (1984). Hepatitis B virus infection: current concepts of chronicity and immunity. *Western J. Med.*, **140**, 754–62

5. Tiollais, P., Pourcel, C and Dejean, A. (1985). The hepatitis B virus. *Nature*, **317**, 489–95

6. Summers, J., Smolec, J. and Snyder, R. (1978). A virus similar to human hepatitis B virus associated with hepatitis and hepatoma in woodchucks. *Proc. Natl. Acad. Sci. USA*, **75**, 4533–7

7. Marion, P. L., Oshiro, L. S., Regnery, D. C., Scullard, G. A. and Robinson, W. S. (1980). A virus in Beechy ground squirrel that is related to hepatitis B virus of humans. *Proc. Natl. Acad. Sci. USA*, **77**, 2941–5

8. Mason, W. S., Seal, G. and Summers, J. (1980). Virus of Pekin ducks with structural and biological relatedness to human hepatitis B virus. *J. Virol.*, **36**, 829–36

9. Szmuness, W. (1978). Hepatocellular carcinoma and hepatitis B virus: Evidence for a causal relationship. *Prog. Med. Virol.*, **24**, 40–69

10. Brechot, C., Pourcel, C., Louise, A., Rain, B. and Tiollais, P. (1980). Presence of integrated hepatitis B virus sequences in cellular DNA of human hepatocellular carcinoma. *Nature*, **286**, 533–5

11. Beasley, R. P., Hwang, L. Y., Lin, C. C. and Chien, C. S. (1981). Hepatocellular carcinoma and hepatitis B virus. A prospective study of 22,707 men in Taiwan. *Lancet*, **2**, 1129–32

12. Brechot, C., Hadchouel, M., Scotto, J., Fonck, M., Potet, F., Vyas, G. N. and Tiollais, P. (1981). State of hepatitis B virus DNA in hepatocytes of patients with hepatitis B surface antigen-positive and -negative liver diseases. *Proc. Natl. Acad. Sci. USA*, **78**, 3906–10

13. Koshy, R., Maupas, P., Mueller, R. and Hofschneider, P. H. (1981). Detection of hepatitis B virus-specific DNA in the genomes of human hepatocellular carcinoma and liver cirrhosis tissues. *J. Gen. Virol.*, **57**, 95–102

14. Shafritz, D. A. and Kew, M. C. (1981). Identification of integrated hepatitis B virus DNA in human hepatocellular carcinomas. *Hepatology*, **1**, 1–8

15. Shafritz, D. A., Shouval, D., Sherman, H. I., Hadziyannis, S. I. and Kew, M. C. (1981). Integration of hepatitis B virus DNA into the genome of liver cells in chronic liver disease and hepatocellular carcinoma. *N. Engl. J. Med.*, **306**, 1067–73

16. Brechot, C., Nalpas, B., Courouce, A.-M., Duhamel, G., Callard, P., Carnot, F., Tiollais, P. and Berthelot, P. (1982). Evidence that hepatitis B virus has a role in liver-cell carcinoma in alcoholic liver disease. *N. Engl. J. Med.*, **306**, 1384–7

17. Okuda, K. and Mackay, I. (eds) (1982). *Hepatocellular Carcinoma*. Technical Report Series, Vol. 74. (Geneva: International Union against Cancer)

18. Popper, H., Gerber, M. A. and Thung, S. N. (1982). The relation of hepatocellular carcinoma to infection with hepatitis B and related viruses in man and animals. *Hepatology*, **2**, 1S–9S
19. Szmuness, W., Alter, H. J. and Maynard, H. E. (eds.) (1982) *Viral Hepatitis*. (Philadelphia: Franklin Institute Press)
20. Dejean, A., Brechot, C., Tiollais, P. and Wain-Hobson, S. (1983). Characterization of integrated hepatitis B viral DNA cloned from a human hepatoma and the hepatoma cell line PLC/PRF/5. *Proc. Natl. Acad. Sci. USA*, **80**, 2505–9
21. Koshy, R., Koch, S., Freytag von Loringhoven, A., Kahmann, R., Murray, K. and Hofschneider, P. H. (1983). Integration of hepatitis B virus DNA: Evidence for integration in the single-stranded gap. *Cell*, **34**, 215–23
22. Kew, M. C. (1984). The possible etiologic role of hepatitis B virus in hepatocellular carcinoma: evidence from Southern Africa. In Chishari, F. V. (ed.) *Advances in Hepatitis Research*, p. 203. (New York: Masson)
23. Shafritz, D. A. and Lieberman, H. M. (1984). The molecular biology of hepatitis B virus. *Ann. Rev. Med.*, **35**, 219–32
24. Vyas, G. N., Dienstag, J. L. and Hoofnagle, J. H. (eds) (1984). *Viral Hepatitis and Liver Disease*. (New York: Grune & Stratton)
25. Blum, H. E., Gerok, W., Tong, M. J. and Vyas, G. N. (1986). Hepatitis B virus infection and hepatocellular carcinoma. *IM* (*Internal Medicine for the Specialist*), **7**, 195–211
26. Dane, D. S., Cameron, C. H. and Briggs, M. (1970). Virus-like particles in serum of patients with Australia antigen associated hepatitis. *Lancet*, **2**, 695–8
27. Almeida, J. D., Rubenstein, D. and Stott, E. J. (1971). New antigen antibody system in Australia antigen positive hepatitis. *Lancet*, **2**, 1225–7
28. Courouce-Pauty, A. M., Plancon, A. and Soulier, J. P. (1983). Distribution of HBsAg subtypes in the world. *Vox Sang.*, **44**, 197–211
29. Stibbe, W. and Gerlich, W. H. (1983). Structural relationships between minor and major proteins of hepatitis B surface antigen. *J. Virol.*, **46**, 626–8
30. Heermann, K. H., Goldmann, U., Schwartz, W., Seyfarth, T., Baumgarten, H. and Gerlich, W. H. (1984). Large surface proteins of hepatitis B virus containing the pre-S sequence. *J. Virol.*, **52**, 396–402
31. Machida, A., Kishimoto, S., Ohnuma, H., Baba, K., Ito, Y., Miyamoto, H., Funatsu, G., Oda, K., Usuda, S., Togami, S., Nakamura, T., Miyakawa, Y., and Mayumi, M. (1984). A polypeptide containing 55 amino acid residues coded by the pre-S region of hepatitis B virus deoxyribonucleic acid bears the receptor for polymerized human as well as chimpanzee albumins. *Gastroenterology*, **86**, 910–18
32. Takahashi, K., Akahana, Y., Gotanda, T., Mishiro, T., Imai, M. and

Mayumi, M. (1979). Demonstration of hepatitis B e antigen in the core of Dane particles. *J. Immunol.*, **122**, 275–9

33. MacKay, P., Lees, J. and Murray, K. (1981). The conversion of hepatitis B core antigen synthesized in E. coli into e antigen. *J. Med. Virol.*, **8**, 237–43

34. Gerlich, W. and Robinson, W. S. (1980). Hepatitis B virus contains protein attached to the 5′ terminus of its complete strand. *Cell*, **21**, 801–9

35. Kaplan, P. M., Greenman, R. L., Gerin, J. L., Purcell, R. H. and Robinson, W. S. (1973). DNA polymerase associated with human hepatitis B antigen. *J. Virol.*, **12**, 995–1005

36. Robinson, W. S. and Greenman, R. L. (1974). DNA polymerase in the core of the human hepatitis B virus candidate. *J. Virol.*, **13**, 1231–6

37. Albin, C. and Robinson, W. S. (1980). Protein kinase activity in hepatitis B virus. *J. Virol.*, **34**, 297–302

38. Robinson, W. S., Clayton, D. A. and Greenman, R. L. (1974). DNA of a human hepatitis B virus candidate. *J. Virol.*, **14**, 384–91

39. Summers, J., O'Connell, A. and Millman, I. (1975). Restriction enzyme cleavage and structure of DNA extracted from Dane particles. *Proc. Natl. Acad. Sci. USA*, **72**, 4597–601

40. Hruska, J. F., Clayton, D. A., Rubenstein, J. L. R. and Robinson, W. S. (1977). Structure of hepatitis B Dane particle DNA before and after DNA polymerase reaction. *J. Virol.*, **21**, 666–72

41. Landers, T. A., Greenberg, H. B. and Robinson, W. S. (1977). Structure of hepatitis B Dane particle DNA and nature of the endogenous DNA polymerase reaction. *J. Virol.*, **23**, 368–76

42. Delius, H., Gough, N. M., Cameron, C. H. and Murray, K. (1983). Structure of the hepatitis B virus genome. *J. Virol.*, **47**, 337–43

43. Charnay, P., Mandart, E., Hampe, A., Fitoussi, F., Tiollais, P. and Galibert, F. (1979). Localization of the viral genome and nucleotide sequence of the gene coding for the major polypeptide of the hepatitis B surface antigen (HBsAg). *Nucl. Acids Res.*, **7**, 335–46

44. Sattler, F. and Robinson, W. S. (1979). Hepatitis B viral DNA molecules have cohesive ends.. *J. Virol.*, **32**, 226–33

45. Siddiqui, A., Sattler, F. and Robinson, W. S. (1979). Restriction endonuclease cleavage map and location of unique features of the DNA of hepatitis B virus, subtype adw_2. *Proc. Natl. Acad. Sci. USA*, **76**, 4664–8

46. Wain-Hobson, S. (1984). Molecular biology of the hepadna viruses. In Chisari, F. V. (ed.) *Advances in Hepatitis Research*, p. 49. (New York: Masson)

47. Galibert, F., Mandart, E., Fitoussi, F., Tiollais, P. and Charnay, P. (1979). Nucleotide sequence of the hepatitis B virus genome (subtype ayw) cloned in E. coli. *Nature*, **281**, 646–50

48. Pasek, M., Goto, T., Gilbert, W., Zink, B., Schaller, H., MacKay, P., Leadbetter, G. and Murray, K. (1979). Hepatitis B virus genes and their expression in E. coli. *Nature,* **282,** 575–9

49. Valenzuela, P., Quiroga, M., Zaldivar, J., Gray, P. and Rutter, W. J. (1980). The nucleotide sequence of the hepatitis B viral genome and the identification of the major polypeptides. In Fields, B., Jaenisch, R. and Fox, C. F. (eds.) *Animal Virus Genetics,* p. 57. (New York: Academic Press)

50. Ono, Y., Onda, H., Sasada, R., Igarashi, K., Sugino, Y. and Nishioka, K. (1983). The complete nucleotide sequence of the cloned hepatitis B virus DNA; subtypes adr and adw. *Nucl. Acids Res.,* **11,** 1747–57

51. Galibert, F., Chen, T. N. and Mandart, E. (1982). Nucleotide sequence of a cloned woodchuck hepatitis virus genome: comparison with the hepatitis B virus sequence. *J. Virol.,* **41,** 51–65

52. Kodama, K., Ogasawara, N., Yoshikawa, H. and Murakami, S. (1985). Nucleotide sequence of a cloned woodchuck hepatitis virus genome: Evolutional relationship between hepadna viruses. *J. Virol.,* **56,** 978–86

53. Mandart, E., Kay, A. and Galibert, F. (1984). Nucleotide sequence of a cloned duck hepatitis B virus genome: comparison with woodchuck and human hepatitis B virus sequences. *J. Virol.,* **49,** 782–92

54. Sprengel, R., Kuhn, C., Will, H. and Schaller, H. (1985). Comparative sequence analysis of duck and human hepatitis B virus genomes. *J. Med. Virol.,* **15,** 323-33

55. Mason, W. S., Aldrich, C., Summers, J. and Taylor, J. M. (1982). Asymmetric replication of duck hepatitis B virus DNA: Free minus-strand DNA.. *Proc. Natl. Acad. Sci. USA,* **79,** 3997–4001

56. Summers, J. and Mason, W. S. (1982). Replication of the genome of a hepatitis B-like virus by reverse transcription of an RNA intermediate. *Cell,* **29,** 403–15

57. Varmus, H. E. (1982). Form and function of retroviral proviruses. *Science,* **216,** 812–20

58. Weiser, B., Ganem, D., Seeger, C. and Varmus, H. E. (1983). Closed circular viral DNA and asymmetrical heterogenous forms in liver from animals infected with ground squirrel hepatitis virus. *J. Virol.,* **48,** 1–9

59. Seeger, C., Ganem, D. and Varmus, H. E. (1986). Biochemical and genetic evidence for the hepatitis B virus replication strategy. *Science,* **232,** 477–84

60. Blum, H. E., Haase, A. T., Harris, J. D., Walker, D. and Vyas, G. N. (1982). Asymmetric replication of hepatitis B virus DNA in human liver: Demonstration of cytoplasmic minus-strand DNA by Southern blot analyses and *in situ* hybridization. *Virology,* **139,** 87–96

61. Fowler, M. J. F., Monjardino, J., Tsiquaye, K. N., Zuckerman, A. J. and Thomas, H. C. (1984). The mechanism of replication of hepatitis B virus: Evidence of asymmetric replication of the two DNA strands. *J. Med. Virol.,* **13,** 83–91

62. Miller, R. H., Tran, C.-T. and Robinson, W. S. (1984). Hepatitis B virus particles of plasma and liver contain viral DNA-RNA hybrid molecules. *Virology*, **139**, 59–63

63. Miller, R. H., Marion, P. L. and Robinson, W. S. (1984). Hepatitis B viral DNA-RNA hybrid molecules in particles from infected liver are converted to viral DNA molecules during an endogenous DNA polymerase reaction. *Virology*, **139**, 64–72

64. Southern, E. M. (1975). Detection of specific sequences among DNA fragments separated by gel electrophoresis. *J. Mol. Biol.*, **98**, 503–17

65. Berninger, M., Hamer, M., Hoyer, B. and Gerin, J. L. (1982). An assay for the detection of the DNA genome of hepatitis B virus in serum. *J. Med. Virol.*, **9**, 57–68

66. Bonino, F., Hoyer, B., Nelson, J., Engle, R., Verme, G. and Gerin, J. L. (1981). Hepatitis B virus DNA in the sera of HBsAg carriers: a marker of active hepatitis B virus replication in the liver. *Hepatology*, **1**, 386–91

67. Lieberman, H. M., LaBreque, D. R., Kew, M. C., Hadziyannis, S. I. and Shafritz, D. A. (1983). Detection of hepatitis B virus DNA directly in human serum by a simplified molecular hybridization test: comparison to HBeAg/anti-HBe status in HBsAg carriers. *Hepatology*, **3**, 285–91

68. Monjardino, J., Fowler, M. J. F., Montano, L., Weller, I., Tsiquaye, K. N., Zuckerman, A. J., Jones, D. M. and Thomas, H. C. (1982). Analysis of hepatitis virus DNA in the liver and serum of HBe antigen positive chimpanzee carriers. *J. Med. Virol.*, **9**, 189–99

69. Scotto, J., Hadchouel, M., Hery, C., Yvart, J., Tiollais, P. and Brechot, C. (1983). Detection of hepatitis B virus DNA in serum by a simple spot hybridization technique: comparison with results for other viral markers. *Hepatology*, **3**, 279–94

70. Brechot, C., Hadchouel, M., Scotto, J., Degos, F., Charnay, P., Trepo, C. and Tiollais, P. (1981). Detection of hepatitis B virus DNA in liver and serum: a direct appraisal of the chronic carrier state. *Lancet*, **2**, 765–8

71. Chu, C.-M., Karayiannis, P., Fowler, M. J. F., Monjardino, J., Liaw, Y.-F. and Thomas, H. C. (1985). Natural history of chronic hepatitis B virus infection in Taiwan: studies of hepatitis B virus DNA in serum. *Hepatology*, **5**, 431–4

72. Krogsgaard, K., Kryger, P., Aldershvile, J., Anderson, P. and Brechot, C. and the Copenhagen Hepatitis Acuta Programme (1985). Hepatitis B virus DNA in serum from patients with acute hepatitis B. *Hepatology*, **5**, 10–13

73. Matsuyama, Y., Omata, M., Yokosuka, O., Imazeki, F., Ho, Y. and Okuda, K. (1985). Discordance of hepatitis B e antigen/antibody and hepatitis B virus deoxyribonucleic acid in serum. *Gastroenterology*, **89**, 1104–8

74. Shafritz, D. A., Lieberman, H. M., Isselbacher, K. J. and Wands, J. R. (1982). Monoclonal radioimmunoassay for hepatitis B surface antigen: Demonstration of hepatitis B virus DNA or related sequences in serum and viral epitopes in immune complexes. *Proc. Natl. Acad. Sci. USA,* **79,** 5675–9

75. Wands, J. R., Lieberman, H. M., Muchmore, E., Isselbacher, K. J. and Shafritz, D. A. (1982). Detection and transmission in chimpanzees of hepatitis B virus-related agents formerly designated 'non-A, non-B' hepatitis. *Proc. Natl. Acad. Sci. USA,* **79,** 7552–6

76. Brechot, C., Degos, F., Lugassy, C., Thiers, V., Zafrani, S., Franco, D., Bismuth, H., Trepo, C., Benhamou, J.-P., Isselbacher, K., Tiollais, P. and Berthelot, P. (1985). Hepatitis B virus DNA in patients with chronic liver disease and negative tests for hepatitis B surface antigen. *N. Engl. J. Med.,* **312,** 270–6

77. Tassapoulos, N. C., Papaevangelou, G. J., Roumelioton-Karayiannis, A., Ticehurst, J. R., Feinstone, S. M. and Purcell, R. H. (1986). Search for hepatitis B virus DNA in sera from patients with acute type B or non-A, non-B hepatitis. *J. Hepatol.,* **2,** 410–18

78. Chen, D.-S., Hoyer, B. H., Nelson, J., Purcell, R. H. and Gerin, J. L. (1982). Detection and properties of hepatitis B viral DNA in liver tissues from patients with hepatocellular carcinoma. *Hepatology,* **2,** 42S–46S

79. Robinson, W. S., Miller, R. H., Klote, L., Marion, P. L. and Lee, S.-C. (1984). Hepatitis B virus and hepatocellular carcinoma. In Vyas, G. N., Dienstag, J. L. and Hoofnagle, J. H. (eds). *Viral Hepatitis and Liver Disease,* p. 245. (New York: Grune & Stratton)

80. Fowler, M. J. F., Greenfield, C., Karayiannis, P., Dunk, A., Lok, A. S. F., Lai, C. L., Yeoh, E. K., Monjardino, J. P., Wankya, B. M. and Thomas, H. C. (1986). Integration of HBV DNA may not be a prerequisite for the maintenance of the state of malignant transformation. *J. Hepatol.,* **2,** 218–29

81. Figus, A., Blum, H. E., Vyas, G. N., De Vergilis, S., Cao, A., Lippi, M., Lai, E. and Balestrieri, A. (1984). Hepatitis B viral nucleotide sequences in non-A, non-B or hepatitis B virus-related chronic liver disease. *Hepatology,* **4,** 364–8

82. Harrison, T. J., Anderson, M. G., Murray-Lyon, I. M. and Zuckerman, A. J. (1986). Hepatitis B virus DNA in the hepatocyte. A series of 160 biopsies. *J. Hepatol.,* **2,** 1–10

83. Romet-Lemonne, J.-L., Elfassi, E., Haseltine, W. A. and Essex, M. (1983). Infection of bone marrow cells by hepatitis B virus. *Lancet,* **2,** 732

84. Romet-Lemonne, J.-L., McLane, M. F., Elfassi, E., Haseltine, W. A., Azocar, J. and Essex, M. (1983). Hepatitis B virus infection in cultured human lymphoblastoid cells. *Science,* **221,** 667–9

85. Elfassi, E., Romet-Lemonne, J.-L., Essex, M., McLane, M. F. and

Haseltine, W. A. (1984). Evidence of extrachromosomal forms of hepatitis B viral DNA in a bone marrow culture obtained from a patient recently infected with hepatitis B virus. *Proc. Natl. Acad. Sci. USA*, **81**, 3526–8

86. Lie-Injo, L. E., Balasegaram, M., Lopez, C. G. and Herrera, A. R. (1983). Hepatitis B virus DNA in liver and white blood cells of patients with hepatoma. *DNA*, **2**, 299–301

87. Pontisso, P., Poon, M. C., Tiollais, P. and Brechot, C. (1984). Detection of hepatitis B virus DNA in human blood mononuclear cells. *Br. Med. J.*, **288**, 1563–6

88. Hoar, D. I., Bowen, T., Matheson, D. and Poon, M. C. (1985). Hepatitis B virus DNA is enriched in polymorphonuclear leukocytes. *Blood*, **66**, 1251–3

89. Morichika, S., Hada, H., Arima, T., Togawa, K., Watanabe, M. and Nagashima, H. (1985). Hepatitis B virus DNA replication in peripheral blood mononuculear cells. *Lancet*, **2**, 1431

90. Dejean, A., Lugassy, C., Zafrani, S., Tiollais, P. and Brechot, C. (1984). Detection of hepatitis B virus DNA in pancreas, kidney and skin of two human carriers of the virus. *J. Gen. Virol.*, **65**, 651–5

91. Korba, B. E., Wells, F., Tennant, B. C., Yoakum, G. H., Purcell, R. H. and Gerin, J. L. (1986). Hepadna virus infection of peripheral blood lymphocytes *in vivo*: Woodchuck and chimpanzee models of viral hepatitis. *J. Virol.*, **58**, 1–8

92. Karayiannis, P., Novick, D. M., Lok, A. S. F., Fowler, M. J. F., Monjardino, J. and Thomas, H. C. (1985). Hepatitis B virus DNA in saliva, urine and seminal fluid of carriers of hepatitis B e antigen. *Br. Med. J.*, **290**, 1853–5

93. Laure, F., Zagury, D., Saimont, A. G., Gallo, R. C., Hahn, B. H. and Brechot, C. (1985). Hepatitis B virus DNA sequences in lymphoid cells from patients AIDS and AIDS-related complex. *Science*, **229**, 561–3

94. Noonan, C. A., Yoffe, B., Mansell, P. W. A., Melnick, J. L. and Hollinger, F. B. (1986). Extrachromosomal sequences of hepatitis B virus DNA in peripheral blood mononuclear cells of acquired immune deficiency syndrome patients. *Proc. Natl. Acad. Sci. USA*, **83**, 5698–702

95. Siddiqui, A. (1983). Hepatitis B virus DNA in Kaposi sarcoma. *Proc. Natl. Acad. Sci USA*, **80**, 4861–4

96. Gowans, E. J., Burrell, C. J., Jilbert, A. R. and Marmion, B. P. (1981). Detection of hepatitis B virus DNA sequences in infected hepatocytes by *in situ* cytohybridization. *J. Med. Virol.*, **8**, 67–78

97. Burrell, C. J., Gowans, E. J., Jilbert, A. R., Lake, J. R. and Marmion, B. P. (1982). Hepatitis B virus DNA detection by *in situ* cytohybridization: implications for viral replication strategy and pathogenesis of chronic hepatitis. *Hepatology*, **2**, 85S–91S

98. Fournier, J.-G., Kessous, A., Brechot, C., Bouteille, M., Tiollais, P. and

Simard, R. (1982). Hepatitis B virus genome expression detected by *in situ* hybridization in PLC/PRF/5 hepatoma cells: relation to cell growth. *Biol. Cell,* **44,** 197–200

99. Fournier, J.-G., Kessous, A., Richer, G., Brechot, C. and Simard, R. (1982). Detection of hepatitis B viral RNAs in human liver tissues by *in situ* hybridization. *Biol. Cell,* **43,** 225–8

100. Gowans, E. J., Burrell, C. J., Jilbert, A. R. and Marmion, B. P. (1983). Patterns of single- and double-stranded hepatitis B virus DNA and viral antigen accumulation in infected liver cells. *J. Gen. Virol.,* **64,** 1229–39

101. Blum, H. E., Stowring, L., Figus, A., Montgomery, C. K., Haase, A. T. and Vyas, G. N. (1983). Detection of hepatitis B virus DNA in hepatocytes, bile duct epithelium and vascular elements by *in situ* hybridization. *Proc. Natl. Acad. Sci. USA,* **80,** 6685–8

102. Blum, H. E. and Vyas, G. N. (1983). Hepatitis B virus in nonhepatocytes. *Lancet,* **2,** 920

103. Blum, H. E., Haase, A. T. and Vyas, G. N. (1984). Molecular pathogenesis of hepatitis B virus infection: simultaneous detection of viral DNA and antigen in paraffin-embedded liver sections. *Lancet,* **2,** 111–15

104. Burrell, C. J., Gowans, E. J., Rowland, R., Hall, P., Jilbert, A. R. and Marmion, B. P. (1984). Correlation between liver histology and markers of hepatitis B virus replication in infected patients: a study by *in situ* hybridization. *Hepatology,* **4,** 20–4

105. Negro, F., Berninger, M., Chiaberge, E., Gugliotta, P., Bussolati, G., Actis, G. C., Rizzetto, M. and Bonino, F. (1985). Detection of HBV DNA by *in situ* hybridization using a biotin-labeled probe. *J. Med. Virol.,* **15,** 373–82

106. Feinman, S. V., Berris, B., Guha, A., Sooknanan, R., Bradley, D. W., Bond, W. W. and Maynard, J. E. (1984). DNA : DNA hybridization method for the diagnosis of hepatitis B infection. *J. Virol. Methods,* **8,** 199–206

107. Hadziyannis, S. J., Lieberman, H. M., Karvountzis, G. G. and Shafritz, D. A. (1983). Analysis of liver disease, nuclear HBcAg, viral replication, and hepatitis B virus DNA in liver and serum of HBeAg vs. anti-HBe positive carriers of hepatitis B virus. *Hepatology,* **3,** 656–62

108. Brechot, C., Bernuan, J., Thiers, V., Dubois, F., Goudeau, A., Rueff, B., Tiollais, P. and Benhamou, J.-P. (1984). Multiplication of hepatitis B virus in fulminant hepatitis B. *Br. Med. J.,* **288,** 270–1

109. Gmelin, K., Theilmann, L., Will, H., Czygan, P., Doerr, H. W. and Kommerell, B. (1985). Determination of HBV DNA by a simplified method of spot hybridization. *Hepatogastroenterology,* **32,** 117–20

110. Shafritz, D. A. and Arias, I. M. (1982). The relationship between infectivity of serum from hepatitis B virus carrier, antiviral therapy, and integrated hepatitis B virus DNA. *Hepatology,* **2,** 106–7

111. Hoofnagle, J. H., Dusheiko, G. M., Schafer, D. F., Jones, E. A., Micetich, K. C., Young, R. C. and Costa, J. (1982). Reactivation of chronic hepatitis B virus infection by cancer chemotherapy. *Ann. Intern. Med.,* **96,** 447–9

112. Hoofnagle, J. H., Hanson, R. G., Minuk, G. Y., Pappas, S. C., Schafer, D. F., Dusheiko, G. M., Straus, S. E., Popper, H. and Jones, E. A. (1984). Randomized controlled trial of adenine arabinoside monophosphate for chronic type B hepatitis. *Gastroenterology,* **86,** 150–7

113. Lok, A. S. F., Weller, I. V. D., Karayiannis, P., Brown, D., Fowler, M. J. F., Monjardino, J., Thomas, H. C. and Sherlock, S. (1984). Thrice weekly lymphoblastoid interferon is effective in inhibiting hepatitis B virus replication. *Liver,* **4,** 45–9

114. Omata, M., Imazeki, F., Yokosuka, D., Ho, Y., Uchiumi, K., Mori, J. and Okuda, K. (1985). Recombinant leukocyte A interferon treatment in patients with chronic hepatitis B virus infection. Pharmacokinetics, tolerance and biologic effects. *Gastroenterology,* **88,** 870–80

115. Nair, P. V., Tong, M. J., Stevenson, D., Roskamp, D. and Boone, C. (1985). Effects of short-term, high-dose prednisone treatment of patients with HBsAg-positive chronic active hepatitis. *Liver,* **5,** 8–12

116. Yokosuka, O., Omata, M., Imazeki, F., Okuda, K. and Summers, J. (1985). Changes of hepatitis B virus DNA in liver and serum caused by recombinant leukocyte interferon treatment: analysis of intrahepatic replicative hepatitis B virus DNA. *Hepatology,* **5,** 728–34

117. Hoofnagle, J. H., Davis, G. L., Pappas, S. C., Hanson, R. G., Peters, M., Avigan, M. I., Waggoner, J. G., Jones, E. A. and Seeff, L. B. (1986). A short course of prednisolone in chronic type B hepatitis. Report of a randomized, double-blind, placebo-controlled trial. *Ann. Intern. Med.,* **104,** 12–17

118. Dooley, J. S., Davis, G. L., Peters, M., Waggoner, J. G., Goodman, Z. and Hoofnagle, J. H. (1986). Pilot study of recombinant human alpha-interferon for chronic tye B hepatitis, *Gastroenterology,* **90,** 150–7

119. Alberti, A., Trevisan, A., Fattovich, G. and Realdi, G. (1984). The role of hepatitis B virus replication and hepatocyte membrane expression in the pathogenesis of HBV-related hepatic damage. In Chisari, F. V. (ed.) *Advances in Hepatitis Research,* p. 34. (New York: Masson)

120. Mondelli, M., Naumov, N. and Eddleston, A. L. W. F. (1984). The immunopathogenesis of liver cell damage in chronic hepatitis B virus infection. In Chisari, F. V. (ed.) *Advances in Hepatitis Research,* p. 144. (New York: Masson)

121. Meyer zum Bueschenfelde, K.-H. and Manns, M. (1984). Immune response to liver membrane antigens in acute and chronic hepatitis. In Chisari, F. V. (ed.) *Advances in Hepatitis Research,* p. 152 (New York: Masson)

122. Dienstag, J. L. (1984). Studies on cell-mediated immunity in chronic

hepatitis B virus infection: elusive goal of virus and host antigen specificity. In Chisari, F. V. (ed.) *Advances in Hepatitis Research*, p. 163. (New York: Masson)
123. Chisari, F. V. (1984). Hepatic immunoregulatory molecules and the pathogenesis of hepatocellular injury in viral hepatitis. In Chisari, F. V. (ed.) *Advances in Hepatitis Research*, p. 168. (New York: Masson)

2

Clinical Value of Serum Bile Acid Determination

G. A. Mannes, F. Stellaard and G. Paumgartner

It has been known for many years that an elevated level of serum bile acids is a highly sensitive and specific indicator of hepatobiliary dysfunction[1] and it seems that serum bile acid levels may give better insight into the functional state of the liver than the traditional liver tests[2,3]. The availability of commercial kits for enzymatic and radio-immunological determination of serum bile acids made it feasible to determine serum bile acids in the routine clinical laboratory and to evaluate their clinical usefulness. For optimal use and interpretation of serum bile acid measurements it is of importance to know the physiological and pathophysiological determinants of serum bile acid levels.

PHYSIOLOGY OF BILE ACIDS

In healthy subjects the bile acid pool of about 6 mmol cycles 5–15 times daily through the enterohepatic circulation. This is accomplished by two physical pumps (gall bladder and small intestine), two chemical pumps (transport system of the hepatocyte and the terminal ileal enterocyte), and two sphincters (sphincter of Oddi and ileocaecal sphincter)[4,5]. The bile acid pool consists of primary, secondary and tertiary bile acids. Primary bile acids are synthesized exclusively in the hepatocyte from cholesterol involving enzymes of the endoplasmatic reticulum, the soluble compartment of the hepatocyte, the mitochondria and the peroxisomes[6,7]. The first step in the formation of bile acids is the 7α-hydroxylation of cholesterol. The 7α-hydroxylase is the rate-limiting enzyme in the biosynthesis of bile acids[8,9]. Subsequently a 3-keto-derivative is formed, which is the precursor of the two main primary bile acids in man: chenodeoxycholic acid and cholic acid. When the side-chain of this intermediate is cleaved after 26-hydroxylation, a propionic acid–CoA intermediate is released and chenodeoxycholic acid, a dihydroxy bile acid, results. Cholic acid, a trihydroxy bile acid, is formed when 12α-hydroxylation precedes cleavage of the side-chain. The rate of cholic acid synthesis is about twice that of chenodeoxycholic acid[10]. Under steady-state conditions daily synthesis of 0.5–1.0 mmol bile acids compensates for faecal loss.

The secondary bile acids are formed in the intestine by bacterial dehydroxylation. Under normal circumstances dehydroxylation starts in the distal section of the ileum and continues throughout the colon. *In vivo* the most frequent reactions are deconjugations and oxidoreductions of hydroxyl groups. The hydroxyl groups, however, differ in their chemical reactivity, the 7α-hydroxyl group being the most and the 12α-hydroxyl group the least reactive one so that 7-oxo-bile acids are formed predominantly[11]. The major secondary bile acids in man are deoxycholic acid and lithocholic acid, dehydroxylation products of cholic acid and chenodeoxycholic acid, respectively. In healthy adults secondary bile acids represent about 20% of the total bile acid pool.

Tertiary bile acids are formed in the liver from secondary bile acids; an example is the formation of ursodeoxycholic acid from 7–ketolithocholic acid[12,13].

Bile acids are secreted by the hepatocyte as conjugates with glycine or taurine, in an average ratio[14] of around 3 to 1. Two lysosomal enzymes, cholyl-CoA-synthetase and acyl-transferase, give rise to this conjugation[14,15]. Conjugation alters the physicochemical and physiological properties of bile acids[16]. The amide bond has an electron-attracting property and increases the ionization of the carboxylic acid group in the glycine conjugates which have a pK of about 3.5. The sulphonic acid group of taurine is intrinsically quite strong (pK 1.5)[17]. At the pH in the gut conjugation increases the hydrophilicity of bile acids and thus decreases their ability to cross the lipophilic layer of cell membranes. As a consequence, conjugated bile acids for the major part are not absorbed passively during their passage through the biliary tree or the small intestine. Most of the intestinal reabsorption of bile acid conjugates therefore occur by an active process in the terminal ileum[18].

After excretion into the gut conjugated bile acids are subjected to deconjugation. The removal of the glycine or taurine conjugate is catalysed by strains of *Clostridium*, *Bacteroides*, *Enterococcus*, and *Lactobacillus*[11,19]. Bacterial modification begins in the distal small intestine; however, most bile acids are absorbed from the small intestine before bacterial deconjugation occurs. Only a small fraction of bile acids escapes absorption in the small intestine and passes into the colon where it is biotransformed by bacteria[11]. The pK of the unconjugated bile acids is higher than the intestinal pH. Consequently free bile acids are mostly non-ionized and are taken up by passive non-ionic diffusion. Trihydroxylated bile acids have a greater affinity to the transport site than dihydroxylated bile acids. The monohydroxylated lithocholic acid has a low solubility. Thus only a minor proportion of lithocholic acid is reabsorbed, contributing only a small fraction to the bile acid pool. In addition to conjugation, sulphation and glucuronidation may occur[20,21]. Sulphation is induced by sulphokinase[22] and glucuronization is carried out by UDP-glucuronyltransferases[23,24]. Conjugation with sulphate and glucuronic acid further increase water-solubility of the glycine and taurine conjugates. Sulphation seems to be the main detoxifying mechanism of lithocholic acid. Sulphate esters contribute 50–80% of total lithocholic acid found in the bile of normal persons[25]. Under certain pathological conditions, especially severe cholestasis due to extrahepatic obstruction, hepatitis, cirrhosis, and tumours of the liver mono-, di-, and trisulphates of bile acids can be identified in the urine and sulphation becomes the main mechanism for elimination of bile acids[21,26,27]. Similarly, glucuronidation of bile acids seems to be an escape mechanism facilitating excretion of bile acids during cholestatic liver injury. In patients with intrahepatic or extrahepatic cholestasis approximately 10–20% of the bile acids excreted in the urine were glucuronic acid conjugates[23]. However, there were considerable individual differences, and in some patients investigated the proportion of the glucuronides exceeded that of the sulphate esters[23]. It has been demonstrated that UDP-glucuronyl-transferases can be induced by barbiturates[28].

The cycling frequency of the bile acid pool is in part modulated by filling and emptying of the gall bladder. During fasting most of the bile acid pool (70–80% at the end of the night) is present in the gall bladder[29]. Gall bladder contraction in response to meals or pharmacological stimuli will increase the hepatic load of bile acids and consequently peripheral serum blood levels of bile acids. Absence of a functioning gall bladder reduces the postprandial rise of serum bile acid levels at least in the first year after surgery[30]. After cholecystectomy the common bile duct can have a certain storage function if the sphincter of Oddi is intact and serum bile acid levels will still raise in the postprandial state although to a smaller extent[5]. The sphincter of Oddi has been supposed to be a regulator of the enterohepatic circulation of bile acids and of bile acid output into the duodenum independently of gallbladder function[31]. After feeding most of the bile acid pool is secreted into the duodenum. The enterohepatic circulation is influenced by the interdigestive intestinal motility which transports the bile acid pool to the terminal ileum. Increased intestinal motility with shortened intestinal transit time stimulates enterohepatic cycling frequency and decreases the size of the bile acid pool, whereas slowing the intestinal transit has an opposite effect[32]. Length and integrity of the small bowel affects the postprandial rise of serum bile acid levels[33,34]. Bacterial overgrowth alters place and rate of bile acid absorption by deconjugation of bile acids[33] and leads to an increase of unconjugated serum bile acids[35].

In healthy subjects the fasting serum bile acid levels of chenodeoxycholic acid and deoxycholic acid are generally higher than those of cholic acid[36]. This is due to the more ready uptake of dihydroxy bile acids compared to cholic acid in the proximal small intestine by passive absorption, and the more efficient hepatic uptake of cholic acid compared to chenodeoxycholic and deoxycholic acid[37-39].

DETERMINANTS OF SERUM BILE ACIDS

Serum bile acid levels at any moment are determined by the instantaneous balance between absorption of bile acids from the intestine and elimination of bile acids by the liver. Hepatic clearance of bile acids occurs during their first hepatic passage from portal blood and after their recirculation from the systemic circulation both from portal and arterial blood. About 80–90% of conjugated trihydroxy bile acids are removed from portal blood during one passage by an active transport mechanism located in the sinusoidal plasma membrane of the hepatocytes. Extraction of unconjugated trihydroxy bile acids is somewhat less, namely about 70%. The values for conjugated and unconjugated dihydroxy bile acids are 70–80% and 50–60%, respectively[40,41]. Spill-over of bile acids into the systemic circulation is the complement of these percentages: about 40–50% of unconjugated bile acids spill into the systemic circulation, whereas only 10–30% of the conjugated bile acids spill over. Despite this spill-over, less than 1% of the exchangeable bile acid pool is present in the blood compartment.

The transport mechanism responsible for hepatocellular bile acid uptake has a large excess capacity. Not only in healthy subjects but also in patients with mild to moderate liver disease, hepatic bile acid transport operates far below saturation[42–44]. Therefore the fraction of bile acids extracted by the liver and its complement, the spill-over into the systemic circulation, remain nearly constant over the whole range of physiological bile acid loads to the liver. Thus intestinal absorption is the major determinant for the diurnal changes of the bile acid levels in peripheral blood. After meals the delivery of bile into the intestine, the flow of bile acids towards the terminal ileum and consequently intestinal absorption and the load of bile acids to the liver, increase. A greater load and a constant extraction fraction result in a greater load of bile acids which spills over into the systemic circulation and leads to the well-documented postprandial increase of serum bile acids. Total serum bile acid levels increases two- to five-fold after a meal[45]. Chenodeoxycholic acid shows the most rapid and largest increase followed by deoxycholic acid and cholic acid. This is mainly due to the fact that chenodeoxycholic acid is absorbed more rapidly from the upper small intestine and is extracted by the liver less efficiently than cholic and deoxycholic acid. The total glycine/taurine ratio of 2.5 in the fasting state increases to a maximum value of 3.3 at $1–1\frac{1}{2}$ hours postprandially and then declines. This shift in glycine/taurine ratio shows that the increase in glycine conjugates exceeds the increase in taurine conjugates in the early postprandial period[45].

CLINICAL APPLICATION OF SERUM BILE ACID MEASUREMENTS

Blood tests are employed in clinical gastroenterology for diagnostic or prognostic purposes. The diagnostic approach is to classify the disease of a patient and implies a binary yes/no answer. For this purpose the bile acid level, a continuous variable, is converted to a discontinuous variable by introducing discrimination limits separating positive from negative results. The prognostic assessment is usually based on an estimate of the severity of the disease when the diagnosis has already been established. Test results are then reported in quantitative terms.

In recent years the results of several studies in larger populations, including healthy subjects and patients affected by various well-documented hepatobiliary diseases, became available. These compare the diagnostic value of serum bile acid levels with that of conventional liver tests in terms of sensitivity, specificity and predictive value. Results on sensitivity and specificity of serum bile acid measurements for detection of liver disease are influenced by the analytical method used. Any method performed by the routine clinical laboratory has to be accurate, sensitive enough to detect bile acids at the picomole level, and simple in handling. Although gas–liquid chromatography with or without mass spectrometry fulfils the first two criteria it is technically too demanding, and thus will remain a research tool. This leaves essentially enzymatic methods and radioimmunoassays for clinical use.

For determination of bile acid concentrations in serum enzymatic methods are widely used and are commercially available[46]. A variety of enzymes specifically cleaving hydroxyl groups in the 3α-, 7α-, or 12α-position are in use[47]. The photometric and fluorimetric assays seem to be rather insensitive.[47] However, sensitivity has been improved by methods using the fluorescence of redox indicators[48]. The recent description of a bioluminescence assay capable of detecting bile acids in the picomole range[49,50] has brought the sensitivity of the assays to the levels of the radioimmunoassays. In addition this method does not require expensive equipment and is quite simple to perform. By incorporating different enzymes into the assay the bioluminescence method also has the potential for measuring individual bile acids.

For sensitive detection in serum many radioimmunoassay techniques, with antibodies against the main bile acids, have been developed. Several of these are commercially available. The potential drawback for the smaller laboratory, namely the need for a liquid scintillation counter or a gamma spectrometer, has been overcome by the development of enzyme-linked immunoassays[51]. Disadvantages of the radioimmunoassays and the enzyme-linked immunoassays are their different specificities and cross-reactivities with other bile acids.

There has been a great deal of controversy as to whether the measurement of postprandial serum bile acids is more sensitive than that of a fasting value for detection of liver disorders. Several studies have shown that the postprandial serum bile acid concentration, which has been called the endogenous bile acid tolerance test, discriminates better between healthy subjects and patients with liver disease than the same measurement in the fasting state[52-54], though not all investigators agree on this point[55,56]. During fasting and after a meal the fraction of bile acids extracted by the liver during one pass should be nearly the same in healthy subjects and in patients with mild to moderate liver disease, because the hepatic uptake of bile acids in these patients is far below its saturation[42,43]. Therefore one could expect similar diagnostic sensitivities of fasting and postprandial serum bile acids.

The conflicting results may be due to differences in the analytical sensitivity and accuracy of the different methods used for bile acid measurements. Consequently Mannes[57] compared fasting and postprandial serum bile acids in patients with cirrhosis of the liver and healthy controls using three methods: an enzymatic assay, a radioimmunoassay, and a gas–liquid chromatographic method. When the enzymatic assay was used the fasting serum bile acid level was a markedly less sensitive parameter (diagnostic sensitivity 79%) for detection of cirrhosis than the postprandial serum bile acid level (93%). When the radioimmunoassay (diagnostic sensitivity 93% for both the fasting and the postprandial state) or an appropriate gas–liquid chromatographic method was used (diagnostic sensitivity fasting 95%, postprandial 93%) fasting serum bile acids were at least as sensitive for detection of cirrhosis as postprandial serum bile acids. Festi[56] has recently shown that fasting serum bile acids are even more sensitive, and discriminate better between normals and patients with liver disease than postprandial serum bile acids. In theory fasting levels are probably more reproducible in the assessment of liver disease since the postprandial rise of bile acids is dependent on a number of highly variable extrahepatic factors such as gastric emptying, digestive hormone release, gall bladder contraction and intestinal motility[58].

Relatively little information is available on specificity, sensitivity and clinical utility of exogenous bile acid loading tests[24,59]. Measurements of oral clearance have proven more sensitive than those of intravenous clearance in the detection of liver disease. This is perhaps explainable by theory: after direct application of bile acids into the vascular compartment the elimination from plasma is highly dependent on liver blood flow, whereas after an oral loading absorbed bile acids are subject to high first-pass extraction and elimination by the liver[41]. For example, when a substance such as a bile acid with a high hepatic extraction of 90% is given intravenously, a 10% reduction in extraction due to liver disease will cause a proportional 10% reduction in plasma clearance; however, if the substance is administered orally and is, like bile acids, nearly completely absorbed, the fraction of the dose reaching peripheral blood from portal blood will be increased from 10% to 20%. By this, a 10% reduction in hepatic extraction increases the spill-over of bile acids by 100%. This explains the disappointing results of intravenous bile acid clearance tests in the detection of liver disease[60].

Bile acid levels are influenced not only by hepatic first-pass elimination, however; they are influenced to a lesser extent also by the clearance of systemically circulating bile acids which reach the liver both via the hepatic artery and via the splanchnic circulation. Decreases in first-pass elimination from portal blood (systemic availability) and reductions of hepatic clearance of bile acids from the systemic circulation contribute to increased serum concentration in patients with liver disease[32]. In accordance with pharmacokinetic principles applied to high extraction compounds it may be assumed that changes in systemic availability and clearance have multiplicative rather than additive effects on serum bile acid levels[61].

DIAGNOSTIC VALUE OF SERUM BILE ACID LEVELS

Important information on sensitivity, specificity and predictive value of serum bile acid levels comes from the study of Ferraris[62]. In the detection of hepatobiliary disease fasting serum bile acids measured fluorimetrically by means of an enzymatic technique (cut-off level 8.4 μmol/l) and aspartate aminotransferase (AST, cut-off 20 mU/ml) exhibited similar sensitivity (78% vs. 74%), specificity (93% vs. 92%), and predictive value for a positive result (94% vs. 93%). Gammaglutamyltranspeptidase (γ-GT, cut-off 28 mU/ml) had a sensitivity of 75%, a specificity of 85% (significantly lower than serum bile acids) and a predictive value for a positive result of 89%. When the predictive value of a positive result, which was obtained in a gastrointestinal unit with a 60% prevalence of hepatobiliary disease, was corrected for the actual prevalence of hepatobiliary disease in the general population (estimated as 1000/100 000) the predictive value decreased to 10% for serum bile acids, to 9% for AST, and to 5% for γ-GT. Since serum bile acids and AST in a mixed group of patients with hepatobiliary disorders have very similar sensitivities, specificities and predictive values, it seems that for cost/effectiveness reasons AST is preferable when a single screening test for liver disease is used. The combination of serum bile acids with AST improves the predictive value of a positive result to 32% vs. 10% of serum bile acids alone in the simulated screening situation with an estimated prevalence of the hepatobiliary disease in the general population of 1%.

When the data of the study of Ferraris[62] are broken down with respect to severity of liver disease, it becomes obvious that γ-GT was found to be more suitable than serum bile acids in detecting mild hepatobiliary disease (sensitivity γ-GT 62%, serum bile acids 48%, AST 49%). However, serum bile acids proved to be significantly more sensitive (93%) than γ-GT (82%), AST (86%), alkaline phosphatase (78%), and other routine liver tests in detecting severe hepatobiliary disease.

Using a highly accurate and specific mass fragmentographic technique Einarsson[36] evaluated the diagnostic value of serum bile acids in anicteric patients with suspected alcoholic liver disease. Whereas serum bile acids showed a high diagnostic sensitivity in cirrhosis of the liver, the measurement of serum bile acids did not discriminate patients with fatty liver from controls. It thus appears that serum bile acid determinations are not useful in the detection of mild liver disorders. Similar results have been presented by other groups using different techniques[56,63,64].

Mishler[65] compared the concentrations of alanine aminotransferase (ALT) and serum bile acids in blood donors and in recipients in whom either non-A, non-B or type B hepatitis developed after transfusion. The results demonstrate that elevated concentrations of ALT in the blood of donors in most instances were accompanied by normal concentrations of serum bile acids.

Should bile acid determination be introduced in clinical practice for diagnostic reasons, it will not be ordered as a single test but rather in combination with other tests of the conventional test battery. Using stepwise discriminant analysis Festi[56] compared a battery of liver tests (AST, ALT, γ–GT, albumin, γ-globulin, bilirubin, alkaline phosphatase, and prothrombin time), serum bile acids and combinations with respect to their capability to correctly allocate subjects into histologically defined groups. The percentage of correct allocations was 75% for conventional liver test battery, 70% for fasting serum bile acids and increased to 80% when conventional liver tests together with serum bile acids were considered. Thus serum bile acids may have diagnostic utility in combination with conventional liver tests because of reducing misclassifications.

CIRRHOSIS OF THE LIVER

It has been shown that patients with advanced cirrhosis of the liver have elevated fasting and/or postprandial bile acid levels in serum. However, in most of these cases serum transaminases and other routine liver function tests will also be abnormal and will point to the presence of liver disease. Patients with cirrhosis and normal transaminases represent a more difficult diagnostic problem, since they may be missed by routine screening tests for liver disease. In patients with cirrhosis of the liver and normal transaminases both fasting and postprandial serum bile acids were abnormal in 93% of the cases, whereas γ-GT (69%), pseudocholinesterase (62%), prothrombin time (62%), γ-globulins (55%), alkaline phosphatase (52%), bilirubin (45%), and albumin (45%) were much less sensitive for the detection of cirrhosis[55].

Fasting serum bile acids were increased in almost all patients (93%) with primary biliary cirrhosis including the sub-group of patients in whom bilirubin is still at normal serum concentration[66]. Patients with normal bile acid levels had early lesions as judged by histological and clinical criteria. With progression of the disease total bile acid levels increased and the ratio of serum cholic to chenodeoxycholic acid decreased.

ACUTE AND CHRONIC HEPATITIS

Several studies to evaluate the value of serum bile acids in the discrimination of chronic active and chronic persistent hepatitis were attempted. Marked overlap between the two types of chronic hepatitis was found by several investigators[3,56,67]. In patients with chronic active hepatitis elevated serum bile acids (measured with a sensitive radioimmunoassay for primary conjugated bile acids) predicted histological evidence of active hepatitis much more reliably than the tests conventionally used for this purpose, such as serum transaminases, bilirubin, alkaline phosphatase and serum proteins[68]. At the time of full remission, serum bile acid levels usually differentiated patients who would remain in remission from those who would subsequently relapse, whereas conventional liver function tests and histological features did not. If elevation of serum bile acids is defined as more than twice the upper limit of normal, elevated levels accurately predicted that relapse would soon follow remission[68].

GILBERT'S SYNDROME

Serum bile acids are a useful adjunct to the diagnosis of Gilbert's syndrome, ruling out occult structural liver disease and confirming the diagnosis of Gilbert's syndrome in the hyperbilirubinaemic patient. Fasting state levels of serum cholyl conjugated bile acids are normal in patients with Gilbert's syndrome, even in the sub-group of patients with metabolic abnormalities in sulphobromophthalein and indocyanine green transport[69-71]. Determination of serum cholyl conjugated bile acids[72] will add a useful, inexpensive and easily performed test to the evaluation of patients with isolated unconjugated hyperbilirubinaemia. The vast majority of patients with structural liver disease of sufficient severity to produce even minimal hyperbilirubinaemia have elevated serum bile acids[69,70]. Because of their high extraction efficiency and resultant sensitivity to disturbances in hepatic blood flow and perfusion, normal bile acids are particularly reassuring in ruling out occult structural liver disease, such as inactive cirrhosis, a condition which may present as unconjugated hyper-bilirubinaemia without other biochemical abnormalities[55,70]. The bile acid concentrations after an oral loading test with chenodeoxycholic acid did not differ from those found in control subjects[73]. Recently an abnormal plasma clearance of orally administered ursodeoxycholic acid was reported in Gilbert's syndrome[74]. In this study urso-deoxycholic acid was administered and measured in the unconjugated form. In contrast to cholyl conjugates, which enter hepatocytes largely via the sodium-coupled transport mechanism[75,76] the hepatic uptake of unconjugated bile acids is less dependent on sodium and may be inhibited by bilirubin[77]. Thus the hepatic uptake mechanism for unconjugated ursodeoxycholic acid differs markedly from that for cholyl or chenyl conjugates[78].

CYSTIC FIBROSIS

Hepatic involvement is common in cystic fibrosis, and cirrhosis gradu-ally develops in a considerable number of cases. Results of standard liver function tests are generally normal, even though liver biopsy may show rather pronounced changes. Though some patients with cystic fibrosis have elevated serum bile acids[79,80], serum bile acid deter-minations seem to be of poor value in evaluating the extent of liver disease in cystic fibrosis[79]. In some cases there may be decreased intestinal input of bile acids because of intestinal involvement in the disease, and this may invalidate serum bile acid levels as a liver test.

PATENCY OF PORTOSYSTEMIC SHUNTS

The serum bile acid elevations before and after portosystemic shunt surgery can be useful in monitoring patency of a shunt[71], since cir-hotics with portacaval shunts have a significantly higher serum bile acid concentration than cirrhotic patients without portacaval shunt[81].

MONITORING OF BILE ACID TREATMENT

In a previous study Whiting[82] predicted the composition of bile acids in bile from that in serum. In chenodeoxycholic acid-treated patients with gall stones a close correlation was found between the serum and biliary proportion of chenodeoxycholic acid. Serum ursodeoxycholic acid also proved to be a very sensitive, specific and convenient means of predicting increased levels of ursodeoxycholic acid in the enterohepatic cycle[83]. These findings suggest that serum bile acids can substitute for biliary bile acids to test patient compliance in bile acid therapy of gall stones.

BILE ACID MALABSORPTION, STAGNANT LOOP SYNDROME

Patients with bile acid malabsorption due to ileal resection have an altered enterohepatic circulation of bile acids with abnormal diurnal profiles of conjugated cholic and chenodeoxycholic acid in serum[84,85]. In comparison to healthy subjects, in patients with bile acid malabsorption, normal gall bladder, and normal liver function the postprandial rise of conjugated cholic acid was smaller and decreased with each successive meal[84], so that the determination of profiles of postprandial conjugated cholic acid levels in serum proved to be a simple and reliable test of bile acid malabsorption[84].

In patients with stagnant loop syndrome abnormally high values of unconjugated and normal values of conjugated serum bile acids have been observed[86]. This is caused by deconjugation of bile acids by micro-organisms within the lumen of the small intestine. Thus the determination of unconjugated bile acids in serum may be of diagnostic value in patients with stagnant loop syndrome[35].

PROGNOSTIC VALUE OF SERUM BILE ACID LEVELS

The prognosis of liver disease can be influenced by many variables, the most important ones being severity and progression of the underlying pathogenic process and functional reserve of the liver. In a prospective study Monroe[3] has found that the degree of serum bile acid elevation reflected histological severity in patients with chronic hepatitis. Fasting and postprandial bile acids were more sensitive than standard liver tests in identifying patients with bridging necrosis or cirrhosis. Serum bile acids have been found to correlate closer with quantitative tests of liver function such as the bromosulphophthalein[2] and indocyanine green clearance tests and the aminopyrin breath test[3] than the conventional tests.

Surprisingly little information is available on the utility of serum bile acid levels as a prognostic index of the mortality risk. In patients with stable alcoholic or posthepatic cirrhosis the concentration of bile acids in serum was more closely correlated with the mortality risk than the commonly used clinical and laboratory parameters such as the portal systemic encephalopathy (graded by the number connection test), ascites, albumin, pseudocholinesterase, bilirubin, prothrombin time, and nutritional state. Serum bile acids alone yielded a prediction of mortality comparable to the Child classification[87]. Measured with a commercial radioimmunoassay for primary conjugated bile acids (Becton Dickinson) fasting serum bile acids below 20 μmol/l indicated a good prognosis. Seven per cent of the patients in this group died within 1 year as compared to 6% of the patients with Child grade A. Serum bile acids exceeding 50 μmol/l were associated with a poor prognosis: 67% died within the follow-up period. This outcome was similar to that of patients graded as Child C, of which 70% died within one year[87]. If serum bile acids and Child criteria were combined by means of a logistic regression analysis, the optimal prediction of prognosis could be achieved with the two parameters serum bile acids and number connection test. These results suggest that serum bile acids alone, or in combination with other parameters, may be a clinically useful prognostic index in patients with cirrhosis of the liver.

References

1. Sherlock, S. and Walshe, V. (1948). Blood cholates in normal subjects and in liver disease. *Clin. Sci.*, **6**, 223–34
2. Grandjean, E. M., Paumgartner, G. and Preisig, R. (1979). Die Gallensäurenkonzentration im Serum nach einer Testmahlzeit bei hepatobiliären Erkrankungen. Ein Vergleich mit quantitativen Tests der Leberfunktion. *Schweiz. Med. Wochenschr.*, **109**, 1280–4
3. Monroe, P. S., Baker, A. L., Schneider, J. F., Krager, P. S., Klein, P. D. and Schoeller, D. (1982). The aminopyrine breath test and serum bile acids reflect histolgic severity in chronic hepatitis. *Hepatology*, **2**, 317–22
4. Hofmann, A. F. (1977). The enterohepatic circulation of bile acids in man. *Clin. Gastroenterol.*, **6**, 3–24
5. Carey, M. C. (1982). The enterohepatic circulation. In Arias, I., Popper, H., Schachter, D. and Shafritz, D. A. (eds). *The Liver: Biology and Pathobiology*, pp. 429–65. (New York: Raven Press)
6. Mitropoulos, K. A. and Myant, N. B. (1969). Conversion of cholesterol

into naturally occurring bile acids in vitro. In Schiff, L. *et al.* (eds), *Bile Salt Metabolism*, pp. 115–26. (Springfield, Il: Thomas)

7. Krisans, S. K., Thompson, S. L., Pena, L. A., Kok, E. and Javitt, N. B. (1985). Bile acid synthesis in rat liver peroxisomes: metabolism of 26-hydroxycholesterol to 3β-hydroxy-5-cholenoic acid. *J. Lipid Res.*, **26**, 1324–32

8. Myant, N. B. and Mitropoulos, K. A. (1977). Cholesterol 7α-hydroxylase. *J. Lipid Res.*, **18**, 135–53

9. Mosbach, E. H. (1972). Hepatic synthesis of bile acids. Biochemical steps and mechanisms of rate control. *Arch. Intern. Med.*, **130**, 478–87

10. Vlahcevic, Z. R., Miller, J. R., Farrar, J. T. and Swell, L. (1971). Kinetics and pool size of primary bile acids in man. *Gastroenterology*, **61**, 85–90

11. Macdonald, I. A., Bokkenheuser, V. D. and Winter, J. (1983). Degradation of steroids in the human gut. *J. Lipid Res.*, **24**, 675–700

12. Hellström, K. and Sjövall, J. (1961). On the origin of lithocholic and ursodeoxycholic acid in man. *Acta Physiol. Scand.*, **51**, 218–23

13. Parquet, M., Metman, E. H., Raizman, A., Rambaud, J. C., Berthaux, N. and Infante, R. (1985). Bioavailability, gastrointestinal transit, solubilization, and faecal excretion of ursodeoxycholic acid in man. *Eur. J. Clin. Invest.*, **15**, 171–8

14. Killenberg, P. G. (1978). Measurement and subcellular distribution of cholyl–CoA synthetase and bile acid CoA amino acid N-acyl-transferase activities in rat liver. *J. Lipid Res.*, **19**, 24–31

15. Sjövall, J. (1960). Bile acids in man under normal and pathological conditions. Bile acids and steroids. *Clin. Chim. Acta*, **5**, 33–42

16. Carey, M. C. (1984). Bile acids and bile salts: ionization and solubility properties. *Hepatology*, **4**, 66S–71S

17. Small, D. M. (1971). The physical chemistry of the cholanic acid. In Nair, P. P. and Kritchevsky, D. (eds). *Bile acids, chemistry, physiology and metabolism*. Vol. 1, pp. 249–356. (New York: Plenum)

18. Lack, L. and Weiner, I. M. (1966). Intestinal bile salt transport: structure activity relationships and other properties. *Am. J. Physiol.*, **210**, 1142–52

19. Macdonald, I. A., Hutchinson, D. M. and Forrest, T. P. (1981). Formation of urso- and ursodeoxycholic acid from primary bile acids by Clostridium absonum. *J. Lipid Res.*, **22**, 652–8

20. Makino, I., Hashimoto, H., Shinozaki, K., Yoshino, K. and Nakagawa, S. (1975). Sulphated and nonsulphated bile acids in urine, serum, and bile of patients with hepatobiliary diseases. *Gastroenterology*, **68**, 545–53

21. Stiehl, A. (1974). Bile salt sulphates in cholestasis. *Eur. J. Clin. Invest.*, **4**, 59–63

22. Chen, L. J., Thaler, M. M. and Golbus, M. S. (1978). Enzymatic sulfation of bile salts. III. Enzymatic sulfation of taurolithocholate in human and guinea pig fetuses and adults. *Life Sci.*, **22**, 1817–20

23. Fröhling, W. and Stiehl, A. (1976). Bile salt glucuronides: identification

and quantitative analysis in the urine of patients with cholestasis. *Eur. J. Clin. Invest.*, **6**, 67–74

24. Matern, S., Haag, M., Homs, C. and Gerok, W. (1977). Oral cholate tolerance test. An application of specific radioimmunoassays for the determination of serum conjugated cholic and deoxycholic acid. In Paumgartner, G. and Stiehl, A. (eds). *Bile Acid Metabolism in Health and Disease*, pp. 253–61. (Lancaster: MTP Press)
25. Palmer, R. H. and Bolt, M. G. (1971). Bile acid sulfates. I. Synthesis of lithocholic acid sulfates and their identification in human bile. *J. Lipid Res.*, **12**, 671–9
26. Stiehl, A., Admirand, W. H. and Thaler, M. M. (1972). The effects of phenobarbital on bile salts and bilirubin in patients with intrahepatic and extrahepatic cholestasis. *N. Engl. J. Med.*, **286**, 858–61
27. Stiehl, A., Thaler, M. M. and Admirand, W. H. (1973). Effects of phenobarbital on bile salt metabolism in cholestasis due to intrahepatic bile duct hypoplasia. *Pediatrics*, **51**, 992–7
28. Bock, K. W. and Fröhling, W. (1973). UDP Glucuronyltransferase activity in isolated perfused rat liver. *Arch. Pharmacol.*, **277**, 103–6
29. Hofmann, A. F. (1983). The enterohepatic circulation of bile acids in health and disease. In Sleisinger, M. H. and Fordtran, J. S. (eds) *Gastrointestinal Disease: Pathophysiology, Diagnosis, Management*, 3rd edn, pp. 115–31. (Philadelphia: Saunders)
30. Ponz de Leon, M., Murphy, G. M. and Dowling, R. H. (1978). Physiological factors influencing serum bile acids levels. *Gut*, 19, 32–9
31. Ashkin, J. R., Lyon, D. T., Shull, S. D., Wagner, C. I. and Soloway, R. D. (1978). Factors affecting delivery of bile to the duodenum in man. *Gastroenterology*, **74**, 560–5
32. La Russo, N. F., Korman, M. G., Hoffman, N. E. and Hofmann, A. F. (1974). Dynamics of the enterohepatic circulation of bile acids. Postprandial serum concentrations of conjugates of cholic acid in healthy, cholecystectomized patients and patients with bile acid malabsorption. *N. Engl. J. Med.*, **291**, 689–92
33. Aldini, R., Roda, A., Festi, D., Mazzella, G., Morselli, A. M., Sama, C., Roda, E., Scopinaro, N. and Barbara, L. (1982). Diagnostic value of serum primary bile acids in detecting bile acid malabsorption. *Gut*, **23**, 829–34
34. Rutgeerts, P., Ghoos, Y. and Vantrappen, G. (1982). Kinetics of primary bile acids in patients with non-operated Crohn's disease. *Eur. J. Clin. Invest.*, **12**, 135–43
35. Setchell, K. D. R., Harrison, D. L. and Gilbert, J. M. (1985). Serum unconjugated bile acids, qualitative and quantitative profiles in ileoresection and bacterial overgrowth. *Clin. Chim. Acta*, **152**, 297–306
36. Einarsson, K., Angelin, B., Björkhem, I. and Glaumann, H. (1985). The diagnostic value of fasting individual serum bile acids in anicteric

alcoholic liver disease: relation to liver morphology. *Hepatology*, **5**, 108–11

37. Angelin, B., Björkhem, I., Einarsson, K. and Ewerth, S. (1982). Hepatic uptake of bile acids in man. Fasting and postprandial concentrations of individual bile acids in portal venous and systemic blood serum. *J. Clin. Invest.*, **70**, 724–31

38. Angelin, B., Einarsson, K. and Hellström, K. (1976). Evidence for the absorption of bile acids in the proximal small intestine of normo- and hyperlipidemic subjects. *Gut*, **17**, 420–6

39. Angelin, B., Björkhem, I. and Einarsson, K. (1978). Individual serum bile acid concentrations in normo- and hyperlipoproteinemia as determined by mass fragmentography: relation to bile acid pool size. *J. Lipid Res.*, **19**, 527–37

40. Marigold, J. H., Bull, H. J., Gilmore, I. T., Coltart, D. J. and Thompson, R. P. H. (1982). Direct measurement of chenodeoxycholic acid and ursodeoxycholic acid in man. *Clin. Sci.*, **63**, 197–203

41. Gilmore, I. T. and Thompson, R. P. H. (1980). Plasma clearance of oral and intravenous cholic acid in subjects with and without chronic liver disease. *Gut*, **21**, 123–7

42. Paré P., Hoefs, J. C. and Ashcavai, M. (1981). Determinants of serum bile acids in chronic liver disease. *Gastroenterology*, **81**, 959–64

43. Poupon, R. Y., Poupon, R. E., Lebrec, D., Le Quernec, L. and Darnis, F. (1981). Mechanisms for reduced hepatic clearance and elevated plasma levels of bile acids in cirrhosis. A study in patients with end-to-side portacaval shunt. *Gastroenterology*, **80**, 1438–44

44. Luey, K. L. and Heaton, K. W. (1979). Bile acid clearance in liver disease. *Gut*, **20**, 1083–7

45. Linnet, K., Kelbaek, H. and Bahnsen, M. (1983). Diagnostic values of fasting and postprandial concentrations in serum of 3α-hydroxy-bile acids and gamma glutamyl transferase in hepatobiliary disease. *Scand. J. Gastroenterol.*, **18**, 49–56

46. Turley, S. D. and Dietschy, J. M. (1978). Re-evaluation of the 3α-hydroxy-steroiddehydrogenase assay for total bile acids in bile. *J. Lipid Res.*, **19**, 924–8

47. Macdonald, I. A., Williams, C. N. and Musial, B. C. (1980). 3α-, 7α-, and 12α-OH group specific enzymic analysis of biliary bile acids: comparison with gas–liquid chromatography. *J. Lipid Res.*, **21**, 381–5

48. Mashige, F., Tanaka, N., Maki, A., Kamei, S. and Yamanaka, M. (1981). Direct spectrophotometry of total bile acids in serum. *Clin. Chem.*, **27**, 1352–6

49. Roda, A., Kricka, L. J., De Luca, M. and Hofmann, A. F. (1982). Bioluminescent measurement of primary bile acids using immobilized 7α-hydroxysteroiddehydrogenase: application to serum bile acids. *J. Lipid Res.*, **23**, 1354–61

50. Schoelmerich, J., van Berge Henegouwen, G. P., Hofmann, A. F. and de Luca, M. (1984). A bioluminescence assay for total 3α-hydroxy bile acids in serum using immobilized enzymes. *Clin. Chim. Acta*, **137**, 21–32

51. Ozaki, S., Tashiro, A., Makino, I., Nakagawa, S. and Yoshizawa, I. (1979). Enzyme-linked immunoassay of ursodeoxycholic acid in serum. *J. Lipid Res.*, **20**, 240–5

52. Fausa, O. (1976). Serum bile acid concentration after a test meal. *Scand. J. Gastroenterol.*, **11**, 229–32

53. Kaplowitz, N., Kok, E. and Javitt, N. B. (1973). Postprandial serum bile acid for the detection of hepatobiliary disease. *J. Am. Med. Assoc.*, **225**, 292–3

54. Barnes, S., Gallo, A., Trash, D. B. and Morris, J. S. (1975). Diagnostic value of serum bile acid estimations in liver disease. *J. Clin. Pathol.*, **28**, 506–9

55. Mannes, G. A., Stellaard, F. and Paumgartner, G. (1982). Increased serum bile acids in cirrhosis with normal transaminases. *Digestion*, **25**, 217–21

56. Festi, D., Labate, A. M. M., Roda, A., Bazzoli, F., Frabboni, R., Rucci, P., Taroni, F., Aldini, R., Roda, E. and Barbara, L. (1983). Diagnostic effectiveness of serum bile acids in liver diseases as evaluated by multivariate statistical methods. *Hepatology*, **3**, 707–13

57. Mannes, G. A., Stellaard, F. and Paumgartner, G. (1987). Diagnostic sensitivity of fasting and postprandial serum bile acids determined by different methods. *Clin. Chim. Acta.* **162**, 147–54

58. Beckett, G. J., Douglas, J. G., Finlayson, N. D. C. and Percy-Robb, I. W. (1981). Differential timing of maximal postprandial concentrations of plasma chenodeoxycholate and cholate: its variability and implications. *Digestion*, **22**, 248–54

59. Miescher, G., Paumgartner, G. and Preisig, R. (1983). Portal-systemic spillover of bile acids: a study of mechanisms using ursodeoxycholic acid. *Eur. J. Clin. Invest.*, **13**, 439–45

60. Thjodleifsson, B., Barnes, S., Chitranukroh, A., Billing, B. H. and Sherlock, S. (1977). Assessment of the plasma disappearance of cholyl-1[14]C-glycine as a test of hepatobiliary disease. *Gut*, **18**, 697–702

61. Neal, E. A., Meffin, P. J., Gregory, P. B. and Blaschke, T. F. (1979). Enhanced bioavailability and decreased clearance of analgesics in patients with cirrhosis. *Gastroenterology*, **77**, 96–100

62. Ferraris, R., Colombatti, G., Fiorentini, M. T., Carosso, R., Arosa W. and de la Pierre, M. D. (1983). Diagnostic value of serum bile acids in routine liver function tests in hepatobiliary diseases. *Dig. Dis. Sci.*, **28**, 129–36

63. Milstein, H. J., Bloomer, J. R. and Klatskin, G. (1976). Serum bile acids in alcoholic liver disease: comparison with histological features of the disease. *Am. J. Dig. Dis.*, **21**, 281–5

64. Tobiasson, P. and Boeryd, B. (1980). Serum cholic acid and cheno-deoxycholic acid conjugates and standard liver function tests in various morphological stages of alcoholic liver disease. *Scand. J. Gastroenterol.*, **15**, 657–63

65. Mishler, J. M., Barbosa, L., Mihalko, L. J. and McCarter, H. (1981). Serum bile acids and alanin aminotransferase concentrations. Comparison of efficacy as indirect means of identifying carriers of non-A non-B hepatitis agents and of onset, severity, and duration of posttransfusions non-A non-B hepatitis in recipients. *J. Am. Med. Assoc.*, **246**, 2340–4

66. Bloomer, J. R., Allen, R. M. and Klatskin, G. (1976). Serum bile acids in primary biliary cirrhosis. *Arch. Intern. Med.*, **136**, 57–61

67. Jones, M. B., Weinstock, S., Koretz, R. L., Lewin, K. J., Higgins J. and Gitnick, G. L. (1981). Clinical value of serum bile acid levels in chronic hepatitis. *Dig. Dis. Sci.*, **26**, 978–83

68. Korman, M. G., Hofmann, A. F. and Summerskill, W. H. J. (1974). Assessment of activity in chronic active liver disease. Serum bile acids compared with conventional tests and histology. *N. Engl. J. Med.*, **290**, 1399–1402

69. Vierling, J. M., Berk, P. D., Hofmann, A. F., Martin, J. F., Wolkoff, A. W. and Scharschmidt, B. F. (1982). Normal fasting-state levels of serum cholyl-conjugated bile acids in Gilbert's syndrome: an aid to the diagnosis. *Hepatology*, **2**, 340–3

70. Douglas, J. G., Beckett, G. J., Nimmo, I. A., Finlayson, N. D. C. and Percy-Robb, I. W. (1981). Bile salt measurements in Gilbert's syndrome. *Eur. J. Clin. Invest.*, **11**, 421–3

71. Javitt, N. B. (1977). Diagnostic value of serum bile acids. *Clin. Gastroenterol.*, **6**, 219–26

72. Simmonds, W. J., Korman, M. G., Go, V. L. W. and Hofmann, A. F. (1973). Radioimmunoassay of conjugated cholyl bile acids in serum. *Gastroenterology*, **65**, 705–11

73. Foberg, U., Fryden, A., Kagedal, B. and Tobiasson, P. (1985). Serum bile acids in Gilbert's syndrome after oral load of chenodeoxycholic acid. *Scand. J. Gastroenterol.*, **20**, 325–9

74. Ohkubo, H., Okuda, K., Iida, S. and Makino, I. (1981). Ursodeoxycholic acid tolerance test in patients with constitutional hyperbilirubinemias and effect of phenobarbital. *Gastroenterology*, **81**, 126–35

75. Reichen, J. and Paumgartner, G. (1976). Uptake of bile acids by the isolated perfused rat liver. *Am. J. Physiol.*, **231**, 734–42

76. Scharschmidt, B. F. and Stephens, J. E. (1981). Transport of sodium, chloride, and taurocholate by cultured rat hepatocytes. *Proc. Natl. Acad. Sci.*, **78**, 986–90

77. Anwer, M. S. and Hegner, D. (1978). Effect of organic anions on bile acid uptake by isolated rat hepatocytes. *Hoppe-Seyler's Z. Physiol. Chem.*, **359**, 1027–30

78. Hill, A., Ross, P. E. and Bouchier, I. A. D. (1983). [125]I radioimmunoassay of serum ursodeoxycholic conjugates. *Clin. Chim. Acta*, **127**, 327–36

79. Strandvik, B. and Samuelson, K. (1985). Fasting serum bile acid levels in relation to liver histopathology in cystic fibrosis. *Scand. J. Gastroenterol.*, **20**, 381–4

80. Davidson, G. P., Corey, M., Morad Hassel, F., Sondheimer, J. M., Crozier, D. and Forstner, G. G. (1980). Immunoassay of serum conjugates of cholic acid in cystic fibrosis. *J. Clin. Pathol.*, **33**, 390–4

81. Poupon, R. E., Poupon, R. Y., Grosdemouge, M. L. and Erlinger, S. (1977). Effect of portacaval shunt on serum bile acid concentration in patients with cirrhosis. *Digestion*, **16**, 138–45

82. Whiting, M. J. and Watts, J. M. (1980). Prediction of the bile acid composition of bile from serum bile acid analysis during gallstone dissolution therapy. *Gastroenterology*, **78**, 220–5

83. Bazzoli, F., Fromm, H., Roda, A., Tunuguntla, A. K., Roda, E., Barbara, L. and Prafulla, A. (1985). Value of serum determinations for prediction of increased ursodeoxycholic and chenodeoxycholic levels in bile. *Dig. Dis. Sci.*, **30**, 650–4

84. La Russo, N. F., Hoffman, N. E., Hofmann, A. F. and Korman, M. G. (1975). Validity and sensitivity of an intravenous bile acid tolerance test in patients with liver disease. *N. Engl. J. Med.*, **292**, 1209–14

85. La Russo, N. F., Hoffman, N. E., Korman, M. G., Hofmann, A. F. and Cowen, A. E. (1978). Determinants of fasting and postprandial serum bile acid levels in healthy man. *Am. J. Dig. Dis.*, **23**, 385–91

86. Lewis, B., Panveliwalla, D., Tabaqchali, S. and Wootton, I. D. P. (1969). Serum bile acids in the stagnant-loop syndrome. *Lancet*, **1**, 219–20

87. Mannes, G. A., Thieme, C., Stellaard, F., Wang, T., Sauerbruch, T. and Paumgartner, G. (1986). Prognostic significance of serum bile acids in patients with cirrhosis of the liver. *Hepatology*, **6**, 50–3

3

Advances in Bile Duct Stone Formation and Dissolution*

H. Wietholtz and S. Matern

INTRODUCTION

Cholelithiasis is one of the most frequent abdominal diseases in North America and Western Europe; 12% of the population are supposed to have gall stones. Most of them are localized in the gall bladder, whereas common bile duct calculi are rare. In autopsy studies cholelithiasis has been found in 6.2–32% of males and in 12.1–57% of females (Table 3.1). The incidence of bile duct calculi varies between 0.5 and 4.5% (Table 3.2).

Choledocholithiasis is a severe disease and complications such as cholangitis, pancreatitis or septicaemia always threaten. Thus a rapid and distinct therapy is required.

This chapter article reviews recent reports on epidemiology and pathogenesis of bile duct stone disease, and deals with one aspect of management, namely dissolution therapy.

EPIDEMIOLOGY OF BILE DUCT STONES

Common bile duct stones originate either from the gall bladder as secondary calculi or are primarily formed in the bile ducts as so-called primary calculi.

* Dedicated to Professor Gerok's 60th birthday

Table 3.1 Frequency of cholelithiasis in necropsy series

Author (Ref.)	Region	Males (%)	Females (%)
Zahor et al.[100]	Malmö	29	52
	Prague	32	52
Torvik and Höivik[2]	Oslo	13.5	28.6
Bateson and Bouchier[3]	Dundee	10.4	23.5
Bainton et al.[4]	South Wales	6.2	12.1
Lindström[5]	Malmö	31.9	57
Massarat et al.[6]	Marburg	22	46
Goebell et al.[7]	Essen	11.1	26.7

Table 3.2 Incidence of choledocholithiasis in three representative autopsy studies

Author (Ref.)	Region	No. of autopsies	Cases with choledocholithiasis	Percentage
Kozoll et al.[8]	Chicago	29 618	146	0.5
Zschoch[9]	Leipzig	34 016	631	1.85
Lindström[5]	Malmö	2 218	100	4.5
Total		65 852	877	1.3

Secondary bile duct stones

Most common bile duct stones are initially formed in the gall bladder. Thereafter they migrate under unknown conditions to the ductal system. This is supported by some observations: about 15% of patients submitted for cholecystectomy simultaneously have bile duct calculi; this is demonstrated in Table 3.3. Bile duct calculi resemble in morphology and chemistry those from the gall bladder[1,17,18].

Simultaneous bile duct stones can be overlooked during surgery. However modern techniques, such as the routine use of intraoperative cholangiography or fibreoptic choledochoscopy, have almost eliminated the problem of undetected retained calculi. Table 3.4 shows that with the improvement of techniques the percentage of retained stones decreased.

Most of the secondary calculi are cholesterol or mixed stones, which are composed of more than 70% of cholesterol[18,26]. Pigment stones containing less than 25% cholesterol[17] are rare in western countries[27].

Table 3.3 Incidence of choledocholithiasis at time of cholecystectomy

Author (Ref.)	No. of operations*	Incidence of choledocholithiasis	Percentage
Glenn and Beil[10]	5797	586	10
Colcock and Perry[11]	1754	139	8
Appleman et al.[12]	4948	480	9.7
Wenckert and Robertson[13]	846	160	19
Moller and Santavirta[14]	1937	250	13
Bartlett[15]	4763	744	15.6
Way et al.[16]	952	137	14.4

* Mainly cholecystectomies; in some cases cholecystostomy

Table 3.4 Incidence of retained bile duct calculi after choledocholithotomy

Author (Ref.)	Year	No. of choledocho- lithotomies	No. of patients with retained calculi	Previous diagnostic procedure
Hicken and McAllister[19]	1964	486	92 (19%)	No operative cholangiography
Hight et al.[20]	1959	77	7 (9%)	Operative cholangiography
Hicken and McAllister[19]	1964	400	44 (11%)	Operative cholangiography
Hicken and McAllister[19]	1964	407	16 (4%)	Repeated operative cholangiography
Fogarty et al.[21]	1968	84	7 (8.3%)	Operative cholangiography
Shore and Shore[22]	1970	100	4 (4%)	Choledochoscopy + operative cholangiography
Longland[23]	1973	37	2 (5.4%)	Choledochoscopy
Leslie[24]	1974	91	0	Choledochoscopy
Finnis and Rowntree[25]	1977	81	0	Choledochoscopy

However in Japan the proportion of patients with pigment stones approaches 70% in rural localities[28] but is decreasing in urban areas where cholesterol stones predominate[29].

Primary bile duct stones

Primary choledocholithiasis is uncommon in western areas. Little, and controversial, information is given about frequencies. Data on incidence of gall bladder stones and simultaneous primary bile duct stones are virtually unavailable. In cholecystectomized patients, values vary from 4% up to 60% (Table 3.5).

The discrepancy arises from the uncertainty of determining whether the calculi are really primarily formed in the bile ducts or are secondary in origin.

Madden et al.[30] gave the extreme value of 60% of patients assumed to have primary bile duct calculi after cholecystectomy, but this very high incidence is based only upon morphological grounds. Braasch et al.[31] aside from a 2-year asymptomatic interval after cholecystectomy, also took the soft brown stones as criteria for primary stones formed in the bile duct. In 55 clinical and autopsy records of patients with congenital absence of the gall bladder and cystic duct, bile duct calculi were found in 20 patients[32].

In a carefully performed study Saharia[34] established the diagnosis of primary choledocholithiasis by four criteria:

1. the patients had undergone previous cholecystectomy;
2. they had at least a 2-year asymptomatic period following chole-cystectomy;
3. stones found in the common bile duct were soft, easily crushable and light brown;
4. there was no evidence of a long cystic duct remnant or biliary strictures resulting from prior surgery.

Only 30 of 758 patients, i.e. 4%, fulfilled these criteria and were identified as patients with true primary common bile duct stones[34]. Nonetheless it is noteworthy that patients with a gall bladder in place, who develop a primary common duct stone, will be excluded by these criteria. The frequency of common bile duct stones after sphincter-otomy is given in a study performed by Seiffert et al[35]. In a multicentre

Table 3.5   Incidence of primary bile duct calculi

Author (Ref.)	No. of cases	No. of primary common duct stones	Percentage	Classification criteria
Madden[30]	126	76	60	Morphological criteria by Ashoff's classification
Braasch et al.[31]	94	37	39	Previous cholecystectomy; a 2-year (mean 5.8 years) asymptomatic interval; soft brown stones
Gerwig et al.[32]	55	20	36	Congenital absence of gall bladder and cystic duct
Thurston and McDougall[33]	91	9	10	Cholecystectomy; earthy brown stones
Saharia et al.[34]	758	30	4	Previous cholecystectomy; a 2-year asymptomatic period; earthy brown stones; no biliary stricture

follow-up trial about 6% of papillotomized patients developed common duct stones within a few years. However it is difficult to determine whether the calculi are primarily formed, since the time interval after papillotomy is not given, and 270 of 954 patients had a gall bladder *in situ* at the time of sphincterotomy.

The composition of common bile duct calculi was analysed in patients undergoing cholecystectomy more than 1 year before, and who had no signs of retained stones postoperatively. In more than 50% of the patients calculi were cholesterol-poor with calcium bicarbonate and fatty acid calcium salts as major components[36].

Likewise an Australian group investigated common bile duct stones of 40 patients whose gall bladder was removed at least 1 year previously[18]. Of the 40 patients 25 (62.5%) were found to have cholesterol-type stones and 15 (37.5%) had pigment stones. Patients with pigment common bile duct stones were significantly older than patients with cholesterol common bile duct stones (68 versus 56 years, median) with a greater proportion of males than females (60% versus 28%).

PATHOGENESIS OF BILE DUCT STONES

Most of the simultaneous and retained bile duct stones have cholesterol as a major component. In contrast the recurrent bile duct stones are frequently composed of pigment, especially calcium bilirubinate. The pathogenetic factors which lead to gall stone formation are different for cholesterol and pigment stones respectively.

Bile duct calculi, mainly composed of cholesterol

Investigations into the pathogenesis of cholesterol gall stone disease have been mainly restricted to cholesterol gall bladder stones; but they should also be applicable to cholesterol bile duct calculi, since the latter are considered to be migrated stones.

The formation of cholesterol gall stones depends on three factors: production of lithogenic bile, nucleation and stone growth. Production of cholesterol supersaturated bile is possible by decreased bile acid secretion[37], increased cholesterol secretion[38] or both the secretion of less bile acid and more cholesterol[39]. Cholesterol crystallization is a precondition for the formation of gall stones. It has been suggested that the gall bladder adds a mucous glycoprotein as procrystallization factor in patients with gall stone disease[40]. On the other hand Holzbach and co-workers discovered a protein factor, gained from normal bile, which inhibits nucleation[41]. The nucleation defect might therefore be due to the presence of a pathological nucleating agent or the lack of a physiological antinucleating agent, or a combination of both.

The mechanism by which cholesterol gall stones enlarge is poorly understood. Crystals have an affinity to each other and stones grow by accretion of cholesterol crystals. Impaired gall bladder motility seems to contribute to stone growth[42].

Whether these pathogenetic aspects are totally valid for migrated or retained stones is unknown. Very little information is available on the mechanisms by which cholesterol stones migrate, and how they are modified in composition and size in the common bile duct. Recently a study by Sauerbruch and colleagues revealed that a high rate of presumably migrated calculi had a cholesterol-rich nidus but a cholesterol-poor husk[43].

Bile duct calculi, mainly composed of pigment

Pigment gall stones are classified into two main types based on differences of pathogenesis, chemical composition and morphological features. One is the black stone; the other the 'earthy brown' calcium bilirubinate stone.

Black or pure pigment stones are formed in the gall bladder especially in circumstances of metabolic imbalance such as haemolytic anaemia or liver cirrhosis, from where they may migrate to the common bile duct. They are mainly composed of pigment polymer, probably polymerized bilirubin derivatives[44], calcium phosphate and calcium carbonate[45].

In contrast to the secondary black pigment stone the calcium bilirubinate stone is the typical recurrent or primary bile duct stone. It is composed of calcium bilirubinate, calcium soaps of fatty acids, small amounts of polymer and a small proportion of cholesterol[46].

The pathogenesis of pigment stones is still unclear. The major factor is the appearance of an excess concentration of unconjugated bilirubin in bile conditioned by hydrolysis of conjugated bilirubin either by hepatobiliary endogenous, or by bacterial, β-glucuronidase[47,48]. This is accompanied by increased hydrolysis of lecithin by bacterial phospholipases, which leads to fatty acid calcium soaps[49].

In normal bile there is no enzyme activity of β-glucuronidase. Two substrates have been suggested to inhibit β-glucuronidase activity: bile acids and glucaric acid. Diet can change the levels of glucaric acid, and possibly contributes to pigment stone formation[50].

Besides extensive hydrolysis of conjugated bilirubin the relative increase of calcium may lead to supersaturation of bile with calcium bilirubinate. This can be due to a decrease of calcium buffers. Bile salts serve as important calcium binders. In animal models bile salt concentration is decreased in infected bile. Other potential calcium buffers such as oxalate and citrate might also be metabolized by bacteria[51].

The mechanism for precipitation and enlargement of pigment stones, as well as the polymerization especially of black pigment stones, has been little studied.

Nucleation and accreation of calcium bilirubinate stones may be initiated by binding calcium bilirubinate to a mucoglycoprotein matrix[52]. The condition under which polymerization occurs is unknown. A hypothetical model is that all pigment stones are precipitated as calcium bilirubinate on a mucin glycoprotein matrix. If there is sufficient time, polymerization can occur afterwards and the stone becomes a black pigment stone. If there is bile infection with high β-glucuronidase activity the excess of unconjugated bilirubin leads to rapid precipitation and accretion without having time for polymerization, thus forming calcium bilirubinate stones[53].

Clinically, calcium bilirubinate stones frequently have retained non-absorbable suture material at their centre. This was confirmed by Wosiewitz et al.[36] and Whiting et al[18]. They found that in 30% of patients with presumably primary common bile duct stones the most important cause of stone recurrence after surgery was incrustation of unabsorbed suture material. Likewise, especially in patients from the Orient, parasites (i.e. *Ascaris lumbricoides, Clonorchis sinensis*) or their ova may serve as a nidus for calcium bilirubinate stones[54].

The pathogenesis of primary and secondary bile duct stones is shown in Figs 3.1 and 3.2, respectively.

DISSOLUTION OF BILE DUCT STONES

Aside from surgery, stone extraction techniques via T-tube or papilla Vateri have the greatest success in the treatment of common duct stones. However, dissolution has an important role, especially if stone extraction is unsuccessful.

One of the major problems is that most dissolution media are only cholesterol solubilizers so that most of the cholesterol-poor bile duct calculi would be unaffected.

Many solvents have been tried over the years, e.g. ether[55], chloroform[56], clofibrate[57] or heparin[58,59] but they did not gain widespread use because of doubtful results.

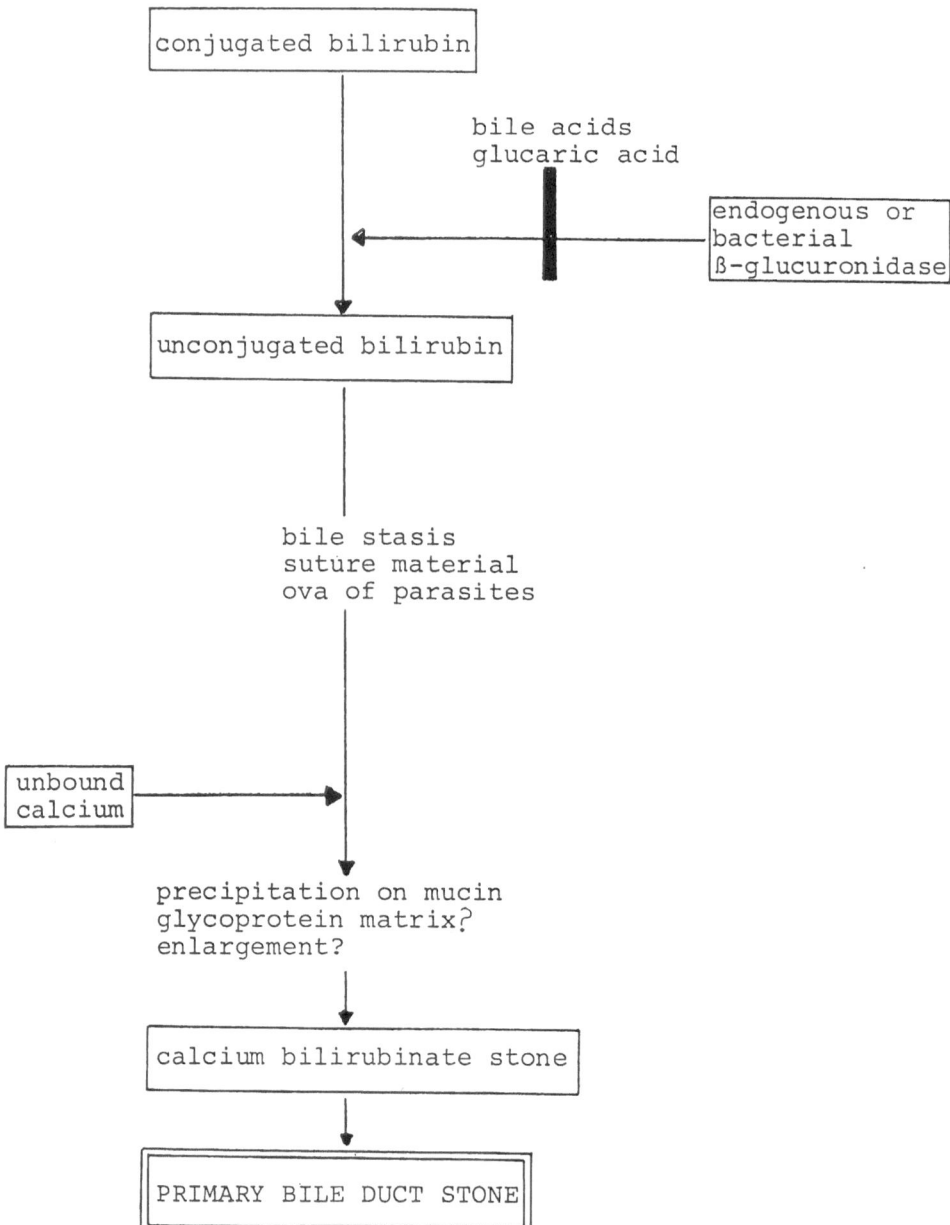

Fig. 3.1 Pathogenesis of Primary Bile Duct Stones

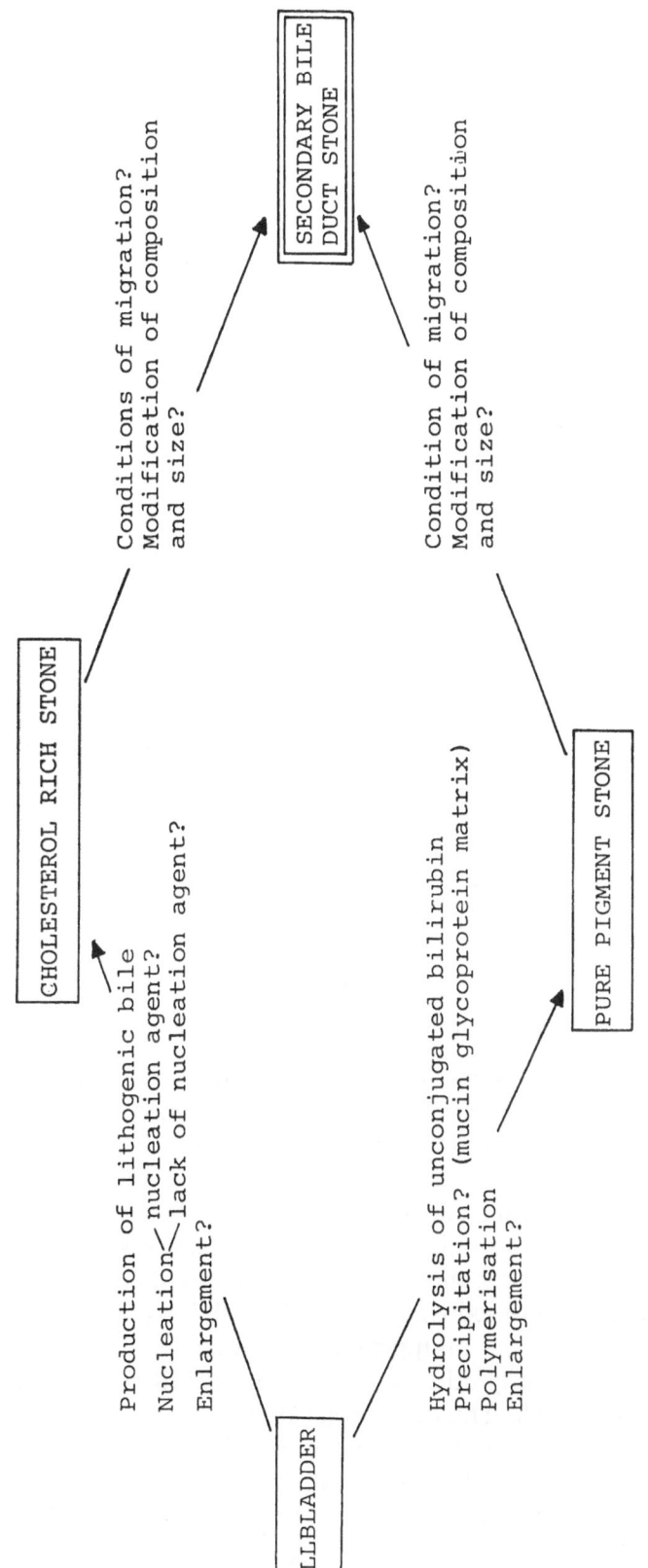

Fig. 3.2 Pathogenesis of Secondary Bile Duct Stones

Dissolution by bile acids

In vitro studies confirm the efficacy of bile salts as cholesterol gall stone solvents[60].

Cholic acid

Bile salt solutions, particularly sodium cholate, were perfused into the biliary tree to dissolve retained common duct stones. Way and co-workers[16] reported a success rate of 55%. Numerous studies followed, with approximately the same success rate. They are listed in Table 3.6.

Cheno- and ursodeoxycholic acid

Successful oral bile salt therapy for retained common bile duct calculi has been reported with chenodeoxycholic acid (see Table 3.7) and ursodeoxycholic acid[73,74]. In the study of Salvioli – a double blind randomized trial – only eight of 28 patients completed the investigation. Not surprisingly the others developed complications and left the study because of biliary pain, cholangitis or surgery. Although the authors established feasibility of oral therapy with a success rate of about 50%, other more rapid techniques which are available are preferable.

Dissolution by mono-octanoin

Mono-octanoin, a medium-chain triglyceride, is a potent cholesterol dissolution agent. In *in vitro* studies weight-matched pairs of gall stones were incubated in 150 mmol/l cholate and mono-octanoin solutions respectively. The rate of dissolution was 2.5-fold in mono-octanoin compared with a cholate solution[75].

Following the *in vitro* studies clinical application was soon reported by Thistle and co-workers. In 12 patients with retained bile duct stones mono-octanoin was infused via T-tube 3–10 ml/h for 4–21 days. In 10 of the 12 patients stone disappearance, or decrease in stone size, occurred[76]. Subsequently other authors confirmed these results; they are listed in Table 3.8. The data reveal that a complete dissolution rate is possible in 55% of all cases, yet 30% do not respond.

In an uncontrolled multicentre trial, which includes in part the

Table 3.6 Dissolution of bile duct calculi by cholic acid

Reference	Year	No. of patients	Application route	No. of stones	Infusion rate (100 mmol/l NaCA)	Treatment duration (days)	Dissolution rate (in no. of patients) complete	partial	overall	Percent	Side effects
Way et al.[16]	1972	22	T-tube	—	30 ml/h	3–14	—	—	12	54.5	Diarrhoea
Lansford et al.[61]	1974	6	T-tube	11	30 ml/h	3–10	5	—	5	83	Diarrhoea, pancreatitis
Britton et al.[62]	1975	7	T-tube	—	30 ml/h	8–12	4	1	5	71	Diarrhoea, nausea, abdominal pain
La Russo et al.[63]	1975	6	T-tube	—	30 ml/h*	—	—	—	2	33.3	Diarrhoea, cholangitis
Iser et al.[64]	1976	14	T-tube	—	30 ml/h	5–14	—	—	5	36	Biliary colic, diarrhoea, dehydration
Christiansen et al.[65]	1978	7	T-tube	—	†	7–10	—	—	3	42.8	Nausea, diarrhoea
Sohrabi et al.[66]	1979	8	T-tube	13	30 ml/h	3–30	—	—	6	75	Nausea, vomiting, abdominal pain
Motson et al.[67]	1981	9	T-tube	—	—	—	—	—	5	55	‡
Total		79							43	55	

* 75–150 mmol/l Na cholate   † Cholate/heparin solution (exact infusion rate not given)   ‡ Not given

Table 3.7 Dissolution of non-obstructive bile duct calculi by chenodeoxycholic acid

Reference	Year	No. of patients	Application route	Daily dose	Treatment duration (months)	Dissolution rate (in no. of patients) complete	partial	overall
Guillet et al.[68]	1976	1	oral	750 mg	12	1	—	1
Barbara[69]	1976	8	oral	2–15 mg/kg	15	3	2	5
Thistle et al.[70]	1978	10	oral	15 mg/kg	>6	—	—	5
Sonnenshein et al.[71]	1980	1	oral	1 g	12	—	—	1
Sue et al.[72]	1981	8	oral	750 mg	4–8	—	—	3

Table 3.8 Dissolution of bile duct calculi by mono-octanoin

Reference	Year	No. of patients	Appln. route (no. of patients)	No. of stones	Stone size (mm)	Infusion rate (ml/h)	Treatment duration (days)
Thistle et al.[76]	1980	12	T-tube (12)	58	5 × 5– 15 × 30	3–10	4–21
Witzel et al.[77]	1980	16	T-Tube (6) nasobiliary catheter (10)	—	—	7.5	6–25
Wurbs et al.[78]	1980	10	nasobiliary tube (10)	—	—	—	—
Schenk et al.[79]	1980	11	T-tube (6), nasobiliary catheter (5)	15	4 × 4– 16 × 18	6	2–10
Jarett et al.[80]	1981	24	T-tube (24)	48	4–14*	2–4	3–112
Gadacz et al.[81]	1981	8	T-tube (8)	16	5–15†	3–7	4–12
Mack et al.[82]	1981	20	T-tube (20)	43	—	3–12	1–11
Uribe et al.[83]	1981	12	T-tube (12)	14	8 × 6– 20 × 15	2–10	2–10
Dawson et al.[84]	1982	17	T-tube (12), nasobiliary catheter (5)	—	—	—	—
Venu et al.[85]	1982	9	Nasobiliary catheter (9)	—	—	3–10	until 15
Steinhagen et al.[86]	1983	6	T-tube, catheter in CBD or CD, PTC, chole-cystostomy (2)	—	5–10†	5–10	2–11
Tritapepe et al.[87]	1984	16	T-tube (15) PTC (1)	25	5–15*	3–4	2–23
Teplik et al.[88]	1984	11	T-tube (8), PTC (2) chole-cystostomy (1)	38	7–27.5†	5	12
Total		172		257			

Abbreviations: CBD = common bile duct, CD = cystic duct; PTC = percutaneous transhepatic catheterization

Dissolution rate (no. of patients)			Percent	Side-effects (no. of patients)	No. of stones treated with success			Percent
Complete	Partial	Overall			Complete	Partial	Overall	
5	5	10	83.3	Mild anorexia, emesis, nausea, abdominal discomfort (?)	37	3	40	68.9
12	—	12	75	Nausea, epigastric discomfort (4)	—	—	—	—
6	—	6	60	Nausea, diarrhoea (5)	—	—	—	—
3	3	6	54.5	Nausea, diarrhoea (6), abdominal colic (5)	3	3	6	40
15	5	20	83.3	Diarrhoea (1), biliary pain (3)	35	2	37	77.1
5	—	5	62.5	Abdominal cramps, diarrhoea (?)	8	—	8	50
15	—	15	75	Nausea, vomiting, epigastric discomfort, diarrhoea (?) GOT, AP ↑ (10)	34	—	34	79
6	1	7	58.3	Nausea, vomiting, diarrhoea, abdominal pain (5), gastric ulcer (1), GOT ↑ (1)	6	2	8	66.6
9	1	10	58.8	Not mentioned	—	—	—	—
3	4	7	77.8	Nausea, abdominal discomfort (6), diarrhoea (5)	—	—	—	—
2	2	4	66.7	Vomiting, abdominal pain (5) diarrhoea (1)	—	—	—	—
11	3	14	87.5	Nausea (10), anorexia (2), diarrhoea (1), duodenitis (1)	16	7	23	92
3	6	9	81.8	Amylasaemia (2), AP ↑ (2), GOT (1), bilirubin ↑ (1), epigastric colicky pain (3)	12	16	28	73.7
95	30	125	72	Total	151	33	184	70

* Average stone diameter (range);
† Stone size (range).

patients of Thistle, Mack, Gadacz and Schenk (Table 3.8), 118 patients with retained common or hepatic duct stones were treated with mono-octanoin via T-tube or nasobiliary catheter. Results, though slightly worse, are comparable to those given in Table 3.8. In 45.8% the stones totally disappeared; in 20.3% there was a reduction in number and size; 33.9% of all patients did not respond[89].

In a very recent and most extensive report held in 1984 at the British Society of Gastroenterology, Palmer and Hofmann presented complete records of 343 patients with retained biliary calculi, who were subjected to mono-octanoin infusion therapy by different infusion techniques. These were application of mono-octanoin via T-tube (230 cases), nasobiliary catheter (82 patients), PTC (23 patients) or chole-cystostomy (8 patients). In 26% stones completely disappeared, in 21% they became smaller, in 9% it was believed that mono-octanoin therapy contributed to successful endoscopic therapy; 33% did not respond to therapy and in 9% treatment had to be stopped because of severe side-effects.

In 67% of all cases side-effects occurred such as abdominal pain (36%), nausea (28%), diarrhoea (15%) and cholangitis (8%). Severe side-effects attributed to therapy were septicaemia in four cases, gas-trointestinal haemorrhage in three and pulmonary oedema in one case[90].

Comparing this recent most extensive survey with the results of the multicentre trial[89] and those given in Table 3.8, the efficacy of mono-octanoin seems to be lower than initially presumed. From the view-point of success, including 'partial success', a rate of 50% may be reached.

Dissolution by GMOC–EDTA–BA (glyceryl-mono-octanoate, EDTA, bile acids)

Based upon these experiences, and especially with respect to the com-position of recurrent bile duct stones whose major ingredients are other than cholesterol in 30–50%, Dr Leuschner and co-workers developed a multicomponent solution consisting of bile acids, dis-odium-EDTA, glyceryl-mono-octanoate and carnosin as buffer[91]. The rationale for the use of this mixture is that the EDTA solution will chelaté calcium salts such as calcium bilirubinate and calcium palmitate, and that mono-octanoin and bile acids will solubilize cholesterol. Carnosin is used to buffer the solution to alkaline pH in order to improve the chelating effect of EDTA.

These workers found that the mixture could completely disintegrate a brown pigment gall stone *in vitro* after 36 h of incubation[92]. In a first clinical trial using alternating infusions of mono-octanoin and bile salt–EDTA through a nasobiliary catheter, they achieved a partial or complete dissolution of bile duct stones in 12 of 20 patients[91].

In a second study following the same procedure they had partial or complete success in six of 10 patients[93] and in a third study in 57% of the patients studied[94]. However, since the composition of the gall stones was not ascertained, the interpretation of the role, especially of EDTA, is difficult. Considering the clinical success rates it needs to be proven whether the combined solution offers any advantage over mono-octanoin. Moreover, the *in vitro* experiments of Allen and co-workers[95] in 1983 seem to cast doubt on the superiority of GMOC–BA–EDTA. This group compared glyceryl–mono-octanoin (GMOC), alternating GMOC/bile acid–EDTA solution, unmodified mono-octanoin and mono-octanoin diluted in 10% of water, and its capacity to dissolve gall stones of similar size containing 94% and 40% cholesterol respectively. GMOC offered no advantage over mono-octanoin and alternating GMOC/BA–EDTA was inferior to mono-octanoin alone for both cholesterol and mixed stones[95].

Altogether controversial observations exist, and a conclusive answer is lacking since a controlled clinical trial comparing the efficacy of the different irrigation media has not been performed to date.

Dissolution by MTBE (methyl-tert-butyl ether)

In 1983, in a first report in abstract form, methyl-tert-butyl ether (MTBE) was introduced as a rapid cholesterol gall stone solubilizer *in vitro* and in animal studies[96]. In additional experiments the authors confirmed that MTBE dissolves human cholesterol stones 50 times faster than mono-octanoin. In dogs MTBE dissolved 14 of 15 surgically implanted human cholesterol stones within 4–16 h. No effect was observed upon a pure pigment stone. Minor side-effects such as nausea, hypersalivation and vomiting occurred in two-thirds of the dogs investigated[97].

In a first clinical approach the same group achieved in one patient dissolution of an intrahepatic stone via nasobiliary catheter within 4 h, and in two further patients gall bladder stones were dissolved via transhepatic catheter placement within 7 h. The agent was well tolerated without major side-effects[98].

In a second clinical study performed by an Italian group MTBE was administered via T-tube within 3–8 h in three patients with retained non-obstructive common bile duct stones. MTBE failed to dissolve the calculi, whereas the subsequently instilled mono-octanoin solution induced partial dissolution in one patient and complete dissolution in the other two patients within 21–29 days[99].

Side-effects of MTBE were nausea, somnolence and histological evidence of duodenitis. The authors conclude that MTBE is only efficient in closed environments (such as the gall bladder), where calculi are continuously contacted by the dissolution agent. In fact, studies in a gall bladder and bile duct model showed that stone–solvent contact is a very important factor in achieving an acceptable rate of gall stone dissolution. Because of their physical properties mono-octanoin as well as MTBE float on bile, whereas gall stones sink. Mono-octanoin, but not MTBE, stirred with bile induce sufficient solvent–stone contact and increase dissolution rate. MTBE is most effective if it is excluded from bile and simultaneously stirred[101].

Clearly further experiences are needed to establish the efficacy of MTBE in gall stone disease.

References

1. Madden, J. L., Vanderheyden, L., Kandalaft, S. (1968) The nature and surgical significance of common bile duct stones. *Surg Gyn Obst* **126:** 3–8
2. Torvik, A., Höivik, B. (1960) Gallstones in autopsy series. Incidence, complications, and correlations with carcinoma of the gallbladder. *Acta Chir Scand* **120:** 168–74
3. Bateson, M. C., Bouchier, J. A. D. (1975) Prevalence of gallstones in Dundee: a necropsy study. *Br Med J* **4:** 427–30
4. Bainton, D., Davies, G. T., Evans, K. T., Gravelle, J. H. (1976) Gallbladder disease. Prevalence in a South Wales industrial town. *N Engl J Med* **294:** 1147–9
5. Lindström, C. G. (1977) Frequency of gallstone disease in a well-defined

Swedish population. A prospective necropsy study in Malmö. *Scand J Gastroenterol* **12:** 341–6

6. Massarrat, S., Klingemann, G., Kappert, J., Jaspersen, D., Schmitz-Moormann, P. (1982) Die Häufigkeit der Cholelithiasis im autoptischen Material und ambulanten Krankengut aus Deutschland. *Z Gastroenterol* **20:** 341–5

7. Goebell, H., Rudolph, H. D., Breuer, N., Hartmann, W., Leder, H. D. (1981) Zum Vorkommen von Gallensteinen bei Leberzirrhose. *Z Gastroenterol* **19:** 345–55

8. Kozoll, D. D., Dwyer, G., Meyer, K. (1959) Pathologic correlation of gallstones. *Arch Surg* **79:** 514–36

9. Zschoch, H. (1964) Die Häufigkeit von Gallensteinen und ihre Kombination mit anderen Befunden. *Dtsch Z Verdauungskrkh* **24:** 145–53

10. Glenn, F., Beil, A. R. (1964) Choledocholithiasis demonstrated at 586 operations. *Surg Gyn Obst* **118:** 499–506

11. Colcock, B. P., Perry, B. (1964) Exploration of the common bile duct. *Surg Gyn Obst* **118:** 20

12. Appleman, R. M., Priestley, J. T., Gage, R. P. (1964) Cholelithiasis and choledocholithiasis. *Mayo Clin Proc* **39:** 473

13. Wenckert, A., Robertson, B. (1966) The natural course of gallstone disease. Eleven-year review of 781 nonoperated cases. *Gastroenterology* **50:** 376–81

14. Moller, C., Santavirta, S. (1972) Residual common duct stones. *Acta Chir Scand* **138:** 183

15. Bartlett, M. K. (1972) Retained and recurrent common duct stones. *Am Surg* **38:** 63

16. Way, L. W., Admirand, W. H., Dunphy, J. E. (1972) Management of choledocholithiasis. *Ann Surg* **176:** 347–59

17. Soloway, R. D., Trotman, B. W., Ostrow, J. D. (1977) Pigment gallstones. *Gastroenterology* **72:** 167–82

18. Whiting, M. J., Watts, J. McK. (1986) Chemical composition of common bile duct stones. *Br J Surg* **73:** 229–32

19. Hicken, F. N., McAllister, A. J. (1964) Operative cholangiography as an aid in reducing the incidence of overlooked common bile duct stones: A study of 1293 choledocholithotomies. *Surgery* **55:** 753–8

20. Hight, D., Lingley, J. R., Hurtubise, F. (1959) An evaluation of the operative cholangiogram as a guide to common duct exploration. *Ann Surg* **150:** 1086

21. Fogarty, T. J., Krippaehne, W. M., Dennis, D. L., Fletcher, W. C. (1968) Evaluation of an improved operative technique in common duct surgery. *Am J Surg* **116:** 177

22. Shore, J. M., Shore, E. (1970) Operative biliary endoscopy. Experience with the flexible choledochoscope in 100 consecutive choledocholithotomies. *Am Surg* **171:** 269–78

23. Longland, C. J. (1973) Choledochoscopy in choledocholithiasis. *Br J Surg* **60:** 626–8
24. Leslie, D. (1974) Endoscopy of the bile duct: an evaluation. *Aust NZ J Surg* **44:** 340–2
25. Finnis, D., Rowntree, T. (1977) Choledochoscopy in exploration of the common bile duct. *Br J Surg* **64:** 661–4
26. Trotman, B. W., Ostrow, J. D., Soloway, R. D. (1974) Pigment vs cholesterol cholelithiasis: comparison of stone and bile composition. *Am J Dig Dis* **19:** 585–90
27. Van der Linden, W., Nakayama, F. (1973) Gallstone disease in Sweden versus Japan. Clinical and etiological aspects. *Am J Surg* **125:** 267–72
28. Kameda, H. (1964) Gallstone disease in Japan. A report of 812 cases. *Gastroenterology* **46:** 109–14
29. Nakayama, F., Miyake, H. (1970) Changing state of gallstone disease in Japan. Composition of the stones and treatment of the condition. *Am J Surg* **120:** 794–9
30. Madden, J. L. (1978) Primary common bile duct stones. *World J Surg* **2:** 465–9
31. Braasch, J. W., Roberts Fender, H., Bonneval, M. M. (1980) Refractory primary common bile duct stone disease. *Am J Surg* **139:** 526–30
32. Gerwig, W. H., Countryman, L. K., Gomez, A. C. (1961) Congenital absence of the gallbladder and cystic duct. *Ann Surg* **153:** 113–25
33. Thurston, O. G., McDougall, R. (1976) The effect of hepatic bile on retained common duct stones. *Surg Gyn Obst* **143:** 625–7
34. Saharia, P. C., Zuidema, G. D., Cameron, J. L. (1977) Primary common duct stones. *Ann Surg* **185:** 598
35. Seifert, E., Gail, K., Weismüller, J. (1982) Langzeitresultate nach endoskopischer Sphinkterotomie. *Dtsch med Wschr* **107:** 610–4
36. Wosiewitz, U., Schenk, J., Sabinski, F., Schmack, B. (1983) Investigations on common bile duct stones. *Digestion* **26:** 43–52
37. Shaffer, E. A., Small, D. M. (1977) Biliary lipid secretion in cholesterol stone disease. The effect of cholecystectomy and obesity. *J Clin Invest* **59:** 828–40
38. Valdiviesco, V., Palmer, R., Nervi, F., Covarrubias, C., Severin, C., Antezana, C. (1979) Secretion of biliary lipids in young Chilean women with cholesterol gallstones. *Gut* **20:** 997–1000
39. Grundy, S. M., Metzger, A. L., Adler, R. D. (1972) Mechanisms of lithogenic bile formation in American Indian women with cholesterol gallstones. *J Clin Invest* **51:** 3026–43
40. Taylor, R. D., Harvey, R., Petrunka, C. N., Strasberg, S. M. (1983) Evidence for a low molecular weight nucleating factor in gallbladder bile of cholesterol gallstone patients. *Hepatology* **3:** 318
41. Holzbach, R. T., Kibe, A., Thiel, E., Howell, J. H., Marsh, M., Hermann, R. E. (1984) Biliary proteins. Unique inhibitors of cholesterol crystal nucleation in human gallbladder bile. *J Clin Invest* **73:** 35–45

42. Bouchier, J. A. D. (1983) Biochemistry of gallstone formation. In: Classen, M., Schreiber, H. W. (eds): *Clinics in Gastroenterology* Vol 12, No 1, pp 25–48. W. B. Saunders Comp., London

43. Sauerbruch, T., Stellard, F., Soehendra, N., Paumgartner, G. (1983) Cholesteringehalt von Gallengangssteinen. *Dtsch med Wschr* **108**: 1099–102

44. Carr, S. H., Ostrow, J. D. (1981) Equilibrium swelling of pigment gallstones: evidence for network polymer structure. *Hepatology* **11**: 1657–8

45. Wosiewitz, U., Schroebler, S. (1978) On the chemistry of black pigment stones from the gallbladder. *Clin Chim Acta* **89**: 1–12

46. Hikasa, Y., Nagase, M., Tanimura, H. *et al.* (1980) Epidemiology and etiology of gallstones. *Arch Jpn Chir* **49**: 555–71

47. Maki, T. (1966) Pathogenesis of calcium bilirubinate gallstones. Role of E. coli, β-glucuronidase and coagulation by inorganic ions, polyelectrolytes and agitation. *Ann Surg* **164**: 90–100

48. Masuda, H., Nakayama, F. (1979) Composition of bile pigment in gallstones and bile and their etiological significance. *J Lab Clin Med* **93**: 353–60

49. Robins, S. J., Fasulo, J. M., Patton, G. M. (1982) Lipids of pigment gallstones. *Biochim Biophys Acta* **712**: 21–5

50. Matsushiro, T., Suzuki, N., Sato, T. *et al.* (1977) Effects of diet on glucaric acid concentration in bile and the formation of calcium bilirubinate gallstones. *Gastroenterology* **72**: 630–3

51. Ostrow, J. D. (1969) Absorption by the gallbladder of bile salts, sulfobromophtalein and iodipamide. *J Lab Clin Med* **74**: 482–94

52. Smith, B. F., La Mort, J. T. (1983) Bovine gallbladder mucin binds bilirubin in vitro. *Gastroenterology* **85**: 707–12

53. Ostrow, J. D. (1984) The etiology of pigment gallstones. *Hepatology* **4**: 215S–22S

54. Bennion, L. J., Grundy, S. M. (1975) Risk factors for the development of cholelithiasis in man. *N Engl J Med* **299**: 1161–7, 1221–7

55. Pribram, B. O. C. (1939) Ether treatment of gallstones impacted in the common bile duct. *Lancet* **I**: 1311–3

56. Best, R. R., Rasmussen, J. A., Wilson, C. E. (1953) An evaluation of solutions for fragmentation and dissolution of gallstones and their effect on liver and ductal tissue. *Ann Surg* **138**: 570–81

57. Garcia-Romero, E., Lopez-Cantarero, M., Quesada, A. *et al.* (1979) The non-operative removal of retained common duct stones after biliary surgery with clofibrate. *J Surg Res* **26**: 129–33

58. Ostrowitz, A., Gardner, B. (1970) Studies of bile as a suspending medium and its relationship to gallstone formation. *Surgery* **68**: 329–33

59. Hardie, J. R., Green, M. K., Burnett, W. *et al.* (1977) *In vitro* studies of

gallstone dissolution using bile salt solutions and heparinized saline. *Brit J Surg* **64:** 572–6

60. Earnest, D. E., Admirand, W. H. (1971) The effects of individual bile salts in cholesterol solubilization and gallstone dissolution. *Gastroenterology* **60:** 772

61. Lansford, C., Mehta, S., Kern, F. Jr. (1974) The treatment of retained stones in the common bile duct with sodium cholate infusion. *Gut* **15:** 48–51

62. Britton, D. C., Gill, B. S., Taylor, R. M. R. *et al.* (1975) The removal of retained gallstones from the common bile duct: experience with sodium cholate infusion and the Burhenne catheter. *Brit J Surg* **62:** 520–3

63. La Russo, N. F., Thistle, J. L., Hofmann, A. F. (1975) Treatment of common bile duct stones by intraductal infusion of cholate: a controlled trial. *Gastroenterology* **68:** 932

64. Iser, J. H., Saxton, H., Wiegard, J., Dowling, H. (1976) Efficacy and complications of T-tube cholate infusion in the treatment of retained common bile duct stones. *Gut* **17:** 815–6

65. Christiansen, L. A., Nielson, O. L., Efsen, F. (1978) Non-operative treatment of retained bile duct calculi in patients with an indwelling T-tube. *Brit J Surg* **65:** 581–4

66. Sohrabi, A., Max, M. H., Hershey, C. D. (1979) Cholate sodium infusion for retained common bile duct stones. *Arch Surg* **114:** 1169–72

67. Motson, R. W. (1981) Dissolution of common bile duct stones. *Brit J Surg* **68:** 203–8

68. Guillet, R., Brette, R., Vacca, C., Piulachs, J. (1976) Lithiase résiduelle du cholédoque. *Chirurgie* **102:** 961–6

69. Barbara, L., Roda, E., Roda, A., Sama, C. *et al.* (1976) The medical treatment of cholesterol gallstones: experience with chenodeoxycholic acid. *Digestion* **14:** 209–19

70. Thistle, J. L., Hofmann, A. F., Beverly, J. O., Stephens, D. H. (1978) Chemotherapy for gallstone disease. *Jama* **239:** 1041–6

71. Sonnenshein, M., Siegel, J. H., Rosenthal, W. S. *et al.* (1980) Recurrent choledocholithiasis following cholecystectomy, sphincterotomy and choledochoduodenostomy: successful treatment with chenodeoxycholic acid. *Amer J Med* **69:** 163–5

72. Sue, S. O., Taub, M., Pearlman, B. J. *et al.* (1981) Treatment of choledocholithiasis with oral chenodeoxycholic acid. *Surgery* **90:** 32–4

73. Lirussi, F., Pedrazolli, S., Gerunda, G., Orlando, R., Venuti, M., Nassuato, G. *et al.* (1981) Retained cholesterol intrahepatic bile duct stones: efficacy of high-dose short-term ursodeoxycholic acid administration. *Curr Ther Res* **30:** 775–85

74. Salvioli, G., Salati, R., Lugli, R., Zanni, C. (1983) Medical treatment of biliary duct stones: effect of ursodeoxycholic acid administration. *Gut* **24:** 609–14

75. Thistle, J. L., Carlson, G. L., Hofmann, A. F. *et al.* (1977) Medium chain glycerides rapidly dissolve cholesterol gallstones *in vitro*. *Gastroenterology* **72:** 1141
76. Thistle, J. L., Carlson, G. L., Hofmann, A. F. *et al.* (1980) Monooctanoin, a dissolution agent for retained cholesterol bile duct stones: physical properties and clinical application. *Gastroenterology* **78:** 1016–22
77. Witzel, L., Wiederholt, J., Wolbergs, E. (1980) Dissolution of gallstones by perfusion with Capmul via a catheter introduced endoscopically into the bile duct. *N Engl J Med* **303:** 465
78. Wurbs, D., Phillip, J., Classen, M. (1980) Experiences with the long standing nasobiliary tube in biliary diseases. *Endoscopy* **12:** 219–23
79. Schenk, J., Schmack, B., Rösch, W., Riemann, J. F., Koch, H., Demling, L. (1980) Spülbehandlung von Choledochussteinen mit Octanoat (Capmul 8210). *Dtsch med Wschr* **105:** 917–21
80. Jarett, L. N., Bell, G. D., Balfour, T. W., Knapp, D. R., Rose, D. H. (1981) Intraductal infusion of monooctanoin: experience in 24 patients with retained common duct stones. *Lancet* **I:** 68–70
81. Gadacz, T. H. R. (1981) The effect of monooctanoin on retained common duct stones. *Surgery* **89:** 527–31
82. Mack, E., Patzer, E. M., Crummy, A. B., Hofmann, A. F. *et al.* (1981) Retained biliary tract stones. Non surgical treatment with Capmul 8210, a new cholesterol gallstone dissolution agent. *Arch Surg* **116:** 341–4
83. Uribe, M., Uscanga, L., Farca, S., Sanjurjo, J. L. *et al.* (1981) Dissolution of cholesterol ductal stones in the biliary tree with medium-chain glycerides. *Dig Dis Sci* **26:** 636–40
84. Dawson, J., Cockel, R. (1982) Retained common bile duct stones: monooctanoin or endoscopic sphincterotomy. *Gut* **23:** 906
85. Venu, R. P., Geenen, J. E., Toouli, J., Hogan, W. J. *et al.* (1982) Gallstone dissolution using mono-octanoin infusion through an endoscopically placed nasobiliary catheter. *Am J Gastroenterol* **77:** 227–30
86. Steinhagen, R. M., Pertsemlidis, D. (1983) Monooctanoin dissolution of retained biliary stones in high risk patients. *Am J of Gastroenterol* **78:** 756–60
87. Tritapepe, R., Di Padova, C., Pozzoli, M., Rovagnati, P., Montorsi, W. (1984) The treatment of retained biliary stones with mono-octanoin: report of 16 patients. *Am J of Gastroenterol* **79:** 710–4
88. Teplick, S. T., Haskin, P. H. (1984) Monooctanoin perfusion for in vivo dissolution of biliary stones. *Radiology* **153:** 379–83
89. Hofmann, A. F., Schmack, B., Thistle, J. L., Babayan, V. K. (1981) Clinical experience with monooctanoin for dissolution of bile duct stones. *Dig Dis Sci* **26:** 954–5
90. Palmer, K. R., Hofmann, A. F. (1984) Monooctanoin therapy – combined experience in 343 cases of retained biliary calculi. *Gut* **25:** 1172 (abstr)

91. Leuschner, U., Wurbs, D., Baumgärtel, H. *et al.* (1981) Alternating treatment of common bile duct stones with a modified glyceryl-1-monooctanoate preparation and a bile acid-EDTA solution by nasobiliary tube. *Scand J Gastroenterol* **16:** 497–503

92. Leuschner, U., Baumgärtel, H. (1981) New aspects of conservative treatment of bile duct stones. In: Paumgartner, G., Stiehl, A., Gerok, W. (eds): *Bile acids and lipids,* pp 357–61. (Lancaster, England: MTP Press)

93. Leuschner, U., Baumgärtel, H., Phillip, J., Jessen, K *et al.* (1982) Spül-behandlung und Endoskopie im kombinierten Einsatz bei der Therapie von Gallengangssteinen. *Dtsch med Wschr* **107:** 285–90

94. Leuschner, U., Baumgärtel, H., David, R., Kirchmaier, C. M. *et al.* (1984) Biochemical and morphological investigations of the toxicity of a capmul preparation and a bile salt-EDTA solution in patients with bile duct stones. *Am J Gastroenterol* **79:** 291–8

95. Allen, M. J., Borody, T. J., La Russo, N. F., Thistle, J. L. (1983) Gallstone dissolution – a comparison of solvents for direct biliary perfusion. *Hepatology* **3:** Abstract 45

96. Allen, M. J., May, G. R., Borody, T. J., La Russo, N. F., Thistle, J. L. (1983) Methyl tertiary butyl ether rapidly dissolves gallstones *in vitro* and *in vivo*. *Hepatology* **3:** Abstract 44

97. Allen, M. J., Borody, T. J., Bugliosi, T. F., May, G. R. *et al.* (1985) Cholelitholysis using methyl tertiary butyl ether. *Gastroenterology* **88:** 122–5

98. Allen, M. J., Borody, T. J., Bugliosi, T. F., May, G. R. *et al.* (1985) Rapid dissolution of gallstones by methyl tert-butyl ether. *New Engl J Med* **312:** 217–20

99. Tritapepe, R., Di Padova, C., Di Padova, F. (1985) Methyl tertiary butyl ether fails to dissolve cholesterol retained biliary tract stones. *Hepatology* **5:** 981

100. Zahor, A., Sternby, N. H., Kagan, A., Uemura, K., Vanecek, R., Vichert, A. M. (1974) Frequency of cholelithiasis in Prague and Malmö. An autopsy study. *Scand J Gastroenterol* **9:** 3–7

101. Allen, M. J., Borody, T. J., Thistle, J. L. (1985) *In vitro* dissolution of cholesterol gallstones. A study of factors influencing rate and a comparison of solvents. *Gastroenterology* **89:** 1097–103

4

Lasers in Gastroenterology

G. Lux and Ch. Ell

The principle of light amplification by stimulated emission of radiation (laser) has been known for the past 25 years. In 1960 Theodor Maiman succeeded, with the aid of a ruby laser, in producing monochromatic and coherent electro-magnetic radiation[1].

The development of efficient, flexible light-transmitting fibres along which laser light can be conducted into the hollow cavities of the gastrointestinal tract, without any appreciable transmission losses, made possible the application of the laser in gastroenterological endoscopy.

The methodic development of the 'laser in gastroenterology' was promoted by Silverstein, Washington; Dwyers, Los Angeles; Kiefhaber, Munich; Frühmorgen, Erlangen. On 5 June, 1975 Frühmorgen in Erlangen succeeded in carrying out the first successful endoscopic laser photocoagulation in the gastro-intestinal tract[2].

GENERAL PRINCIPLES OF THE LASER

Laser light is characterized by its monochromaticity, coherence, and high parallelism. These characteristics are achieved through the principle of induced emission of radiation: when electromagnetic radiation (photons) impinges upon excited electrons, the latter are induced to give up photons, the wavelength and phase of which correspond exactly with those of the impinging radiation. In this manner light amplification of the primary photon wave, characterized by mono-

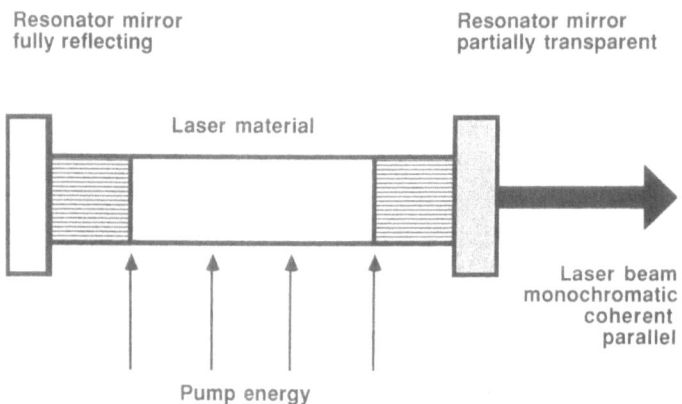

Fig. 4.1   The principle of a laser resonator

chromaticity and coherence, is achieved. The principle of light amplification by the induced emission of radiation may be explained in the
case of the neodymium–YAG laser – a so-called solid state laser –
which can serve as an example (Fig. 4.1). Neodymium atoms, which
are to be excited for subsequent photoemission, are contained within
an yttrium–aluminium garnet crystal. This latter, the so-called laser
rod, is arranged along the longitudinal axis of an elliptical resonator.
In order to excite the active laser medium, energy must be applied
from outside – so-called optical pumping. In the case of the neodymium–YAG laser this is achieved with the aid of high-power-density
krypton or iodine–tungsten lamps. On plane-parallel sides of the
resonator housing at each end of the laser rod, mirrors are arranged,
one reflecting almost completely (99% reflectivity), the other being
semi-transparent. Optical pumping stimulates the electrons of some
of the atoms to move up to a higher energy level. Some electrons drop
back spontaneously into the ground state, emitting radiation while
doing so – part of which is lost in the form of lateral scattering. Some
of the photons are emitted along the axis of the laser rod, and reflected
by one of the two mirrors; on their return journey they are either
absorbed or cause excited atoms to emit a photon. When, on passage
of the light wave through the laser medium, more than 50% of the
neodymium atoms are in an excited state, more photons are liberated
by stimulated emission than are absorbed by non-excited atoms.

With a suitable distance between the mirrors the continued reflection of the light between them leads to the production of a stationary wave which, as a result of the constant supply of energy through pumping represents an additional increase in light amplification. If required, a given portion of the laser light can be 'coupled out', focused by means of a system of lenses, and then transmitted via a flexible quartz fibre to the site of application[3, 4].

LASER SYSTEMS

In accordance with the physical state of the active laser medium, a differentiation is made between solid-state lasers (e.g. neodymium–YAG laser, ruby laser), liquid lasers (e.g. dye lasers), and gas lasers (e.g. argon laser, CO_2 laser).

The laser systems presently used in medicine are designed predominantly for continuous operation. The power output delivered is between 10^{-3} and 10^2 watts.

An increase in power output over a short period can be achieved by pulsed laser operation. The simplest method for producing short light pulses of high power density is to pulse the excitation energy of the laser (optical pumping). In this manner, power outputs of 10^2 to 10^5 watts can be achieved for periods of 10^{-2} to 10^{-6} seconds (Fig. 4.1).

A further principle, the Q-switched laser, is as follows: with continuous optical pumping, maximum excitation energy is stored within the laser crystal, and is emitted in the form of a very short high-intensity pulse of light. Q-switched laser systems are capable of producing output powers of 10^6 watts, at a pulse duration of up to 10^{-9} seconds (for further details see Refs 5 and 6).

LASER-INDUCED PHOTOPHYSICAL PROCESSES

The nature and extent of photophysical processes induced by laser light are determined by the following parameters:

1. the physical parameters of the radiation (wavelength, exposure time, output and energy density);
2. optical parameters (reflection, scattering, transmission and absorption);

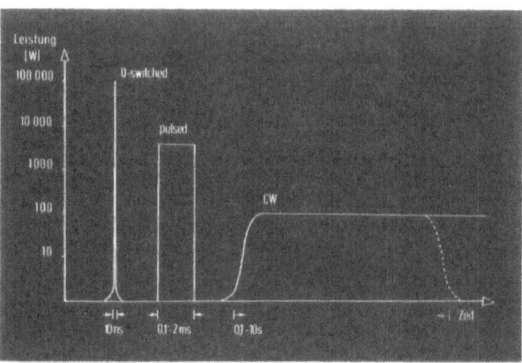

Fig. 4.2 Continuous-wave laser and pulsed laser: principle of radiation; *y*-axis: energy, *x*-axis: time

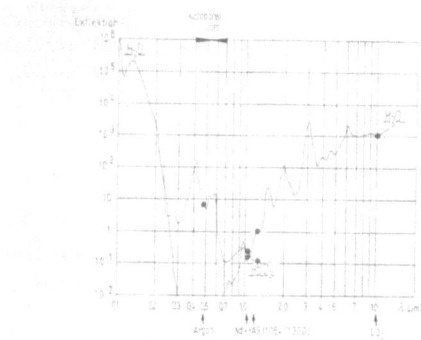

Fig. 4.3 Extinction rate of H_2O, hemoglobin and melanin; ↑argon-laser; ↑↑Nd:YAG laser

3. thermal parameters (thermal conductivity, specific heat and the local diffusion rate of the tissue).

Four major physical processes can be differentiated[7]. Most commonly known is the *thermal effect* of laser light (Fig. 4.2). Irreversible tissue damage with denaturation of protein occurs at temperatures of about 60 °C. Between 90 °C and 100 °C tissue water begins to boil. At higher temperatures charring takes place. The black carbon on the tissue surface increases absorption; if the application of laser energy is continued the temperature can rapidly rise to several hundred degrees, or even exceed 1000 °C, resulting in melting, burning and, finally vaporization of all chemical compounds[8].

Chemical processes are induced at extremely low energy densities and relatively long exposure times. By combining photosensitizing substances and the appropriate laser light, cytotoxic processes can be induced selectively[9, 10]. The third photophysical principle is the *conversion of light energy into mechanical energy* (electromechanical effect). The optical breakdown required for this is characterized by the stages of plasma formation, plasma expansion, and the development of a shock wave. These effects can be achieved with Q-switched laser systems only[11], providing extremely high energy densities at the focus of the laser. So far, little is known about the significance of the so-called *photoablative laser effect*. Excimer lasers operating in the ultraviolet range can produce energy densities between those of Q-switched and those of the continuous-wave lasers by pulsed mode. With exposure times in the nanosecond range, non-thermal tissue-destroying or tissue-ablating effects can be achieved through the selective breakdown of intramolecular bonds (photodissociation)[12, 13].

LASER SYSTEMS IN GASTROENTEROLOGY

At the present time the system preferred by most gastroenterologists is the neodymium–YAG laser. Today, argon and carbon dioxide lasers are of little importance. If the absorption spectra of haemoglobin (blood) and water (water-containing tissue), are compared, the different effects of the various laser systems can be understood (Table 4.1; Fig. 4.3). With its wavelength of $478\,\mu m$ – close to the absorption maximum of haemoglobin – the argon laser is highly suitable for haemostasis and coagulation. At a wavelength of $10\,600\,nm$ – the CO_2 laser – maximum absorption of light occurs in water, causing vaporization of the water content and disruption of the tissue. Utilizing this principle the carbon dioxide laser may be called a 'laser scalpel'[14]. Both argon and carbon dioxide laser light is primarily absorbed at the surface of the tissue with a low depth of penetration. In contrast to these two laser systems, the depth of penetration of the neodymium–YAG laser is relatively high, since the absorption of light by organic material in the near-infrared range at 1064 nm is small, while transmission in water is high. For this reason the optical parameter of light scattering is of importance here. At low output powers (30–40 watts), a homogeneous distribution of the radiation within the tissue occurs,

Table 4.1 Relationship between temperature and tissue event (according to Ref. 33)

Critical temperature (°C)	Histological event	Endoscopic manifestation
45	Cell death, oedema endothelial damage, vasodilatation	Erythema, oedema cuff
60	Protein coagulates	Tissue turns grey–brown, blood turns black
80	Denatured collagen contracts, blood vessels constrict	Tissue 'puckers'
100	Tissue water boils	Vaporization causes a divot
210 +	Dehydrated tissue burns	Blackened tissue disappears ± glowing embers

causing homogeneous coagulation necrosis. At higher powers (80–100 watts), vaporization effects are obtained[7, 15]. Argon and pumped dye lasers with a wavelength of 630 nm are already being used for photodynamic therapy[10, 16]. The utilization of the phenomenon of autofluorescence of photosensitized tumours exposed to a wavelength of 407 nm (krypton laser) makes selective tumour diagnosis possible, at least experimentally. However, there are problems such as making the autofluorescence visible, and there is limited documentation on the tumour-destroying effect and tumour cell selectivity. The future role of laser diagnosis and therapy with photosensitizing substances still needs evaluation in the field of gastroenterology. Furthermore the photosensitizing substances presently available are associated with major systemic side-effects[17].

At the present time basic experiments are necessary to evaluate the possible role of different kinds of laser systems: neodymium–YAG laser systems with a wavelength of 1320 nm for tumour therapy, pulsed neodymium–YAG and pulsed dye lasers for lithotripsy and treatment of oesophageal varices, and the so-called excimer laser for tumour destruction and/or lithotripsy.

ENERGY TRANSMISSION – ENERGY APPLICATION

In all laser systems employed in gastroenterology the transmission of energy is effected through a flexible quartz fibre[18] enclosed within a Teflon sheath to protect against fracture. The neodymium–YAG laser (wavelength 1064 nm), is usually transmitted through a fibre with a diameter of 0.6 mm. The tip of the fibre is bathed in a constant flow of carbon dioxide to prevent its contamination with fluids and necrotic tissue, and thus its self-destruction by burning.

For the application of light energy the non-contact method has proved of value. The distance between the tip of the fibre and the tissue to be treated is 3–10 mm. A pilot light (helium–neon laser) is employed to facilitate aiming[8].

Recently the contact method of laser treatment using sapphire tips has been recommended. An advantage of the contact method might be that less energy is needed to achieve identical effects, i.e. one-third to one-quarter of the energy has to be applied due to the higher energy density and the smaller loss of energy by backscattering. In the case of the non-contact method the loss of energy can be as much as 40%. Using sapphire tips, the tissue-damaging effect can be accurately calculated and estimated. With the non-contact method the distance between the tip of the fibre and the tissue varies, and thus also the energy density effective in the tissue. The use of water irrigation eliminates the need for gas insufflation, which is painful for the patient.

A further variation of the contact method applies a 'naked' quartz fibre without insulation at the distal tip directly to the tissue. A continuous flow of gas can be avoided, and destruction of the tip of the fibre is accepted[20].

At the present time there are only a few applications for the contact method, such as total tumour stenosis, over-growth of an endo-prosthesis with tumour tissue, and high-grade stenoses in the large bowel.

ABLATIVE LASER THERAPY

One prerequisite for the development of operative endoscopy was cutting and coagulating by high-frequency diathermy. In principle, high-frequency diathermy can be replaced in all its fields of application by the laser beam. The question must be asked, however, whether this will result in advantages or disadvantages in respect to diagnosis, complications or economic aspects.

The ability of the laser to vaporize or coagulate tissue opens up the possibility of removing, either completely or partially, benign or malignant neoplasias within the gastro-intestinal tract. In addition to these theoretical considerations, ablative laser therapy is also based on practical experience with laser treatment of bleeding tumours and of tumour stenoses, since here, apart from the desired effect of haemostasis, the removal of neoplastic tissue and/or the re-canalization of tumour stenoses proved feasible. The first attempts at treating gastrointestinal tumours and tumour stenoses with the laser[21-23] were made long after it had been demonstrated that the laser was capable of ablating tumour tissue[29]. Subsequently, further results of palliative laser therapy in tumours of the upper gastrointestinal tract were published[19-23, 25-41].

Palliative tumour therapy

Tumour stenoses of the upper gastrointestinal tract

By the time the diagnosis is established, slightly less than one-half of the patients with oesophageal carcinoma are no longer operable[42]. Similar figures apply for carcinoma of the cardiac region.

The cardinal symptom of tumour stenosis of the upper digestive tract is dysphagia with the sequential loss of weight, malnutrition, aspiration and, not infrequently, social isolation, often associated with frequent periods of hospitalization. Thus the objective of palliative therapy is the 'normalization of the patient's life' by enabling him to swallow food and saliva. Bleeding from tumours of the upper gastrointestinal tract is far less frequently seen. An increase in the survival rate is not to be expected from local measures such as laser coagulation.

Applications for endoscopic laser palliation are tumour stenoses of the upper gastrointestinal (GI) tract caused mainly by oesophageal and gastric carcinoma, and anastomotic recurrences after resection of oesophageal or gastric tumours. A prerequisite for palliative laser therapy is local or general inoperability, which has to be established unequivocally by preoperative procedures; otherwise explorative surgery has to be performed. In the case of bleeding from tumours of the upper GI tract, laser haemostasis is also employed in the case of operable patients.

Laser therapy is not applicable to oesophago-bronchial or oeso-phago-mediastinal fistulae.

Materials and method As already mentioned, the powerful neo-dymium–YAG laser (wavelength 1064 nm), which is suitable both for coagulation and vaporization of tumour tissue, has become generally accepted. The power output required to treat tumours in the upper gastrointestinal tract is between 80 and 100 watts. Individual reports on tumour destruction via coagulation necrosis induced by an argon laser are mainly of historical interest[43, 44]. Photodynamic treatment with the aid of argon-pumped dye lasers and hematoporphyrin deri-vates (HpD) is still in its early stages, and this form of treatment is more likely to be suitable for the curative therapy of small malignancies rather than for palliative tumour treatment[10, 45].

Contact-free application of laser energy is generally accepted. Only when inflammable material such as bridging tubes might be exposed to the laser beam is the contact method to be recommended. Most authors prefer the flexible quartz fibre as transmission system (MBB, Munich). The fibre is kept clear of blood and necrotic tissue by a constant flow of CO_2. The divergence angle of 10° of the emitted laser beam permits the distance between the tumour and the tip of the fibre to be varied between 3 and 10 mm. The three-channel endoscope (TGF1DL Olympus, Tokyo) with an integrated triconical quartz fibre (divergence angle 4.2°) as originally described by Nath[18], is less fre-quently used. The latter system does not need a constant flow of gas.

Most authors prefer to use routine gastroscopes, for example GIFQ$_{10}$ or GFXQ$_{10}$ (Olympus, Tokyo), while others prefer oblique optics (GIFK$_{10}$, Olympus, Tokyo) or those with two working channels. Since laser energy reflected by the tissue can damage the tip of the instrument, endoscopes with laser-resistant tips should be used. The latter are of white colour and of various materials (Teflon, ceramic).

The first reports on palliative laser therapy[21-23, 31, 32, 41], recommended starting at the proximal end of the tumour (Fig. 4.4). The laser beam is guided concentrically around the luminal opening while widening

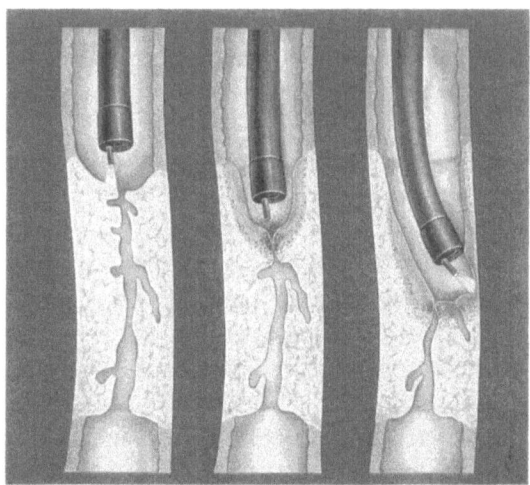

Fig. 4.4   Laser therapy beginning at the proximal margin with stepwise progression to the distal parts, in the middle part correct axis, in the right part 'via falsa' with danger of perforation

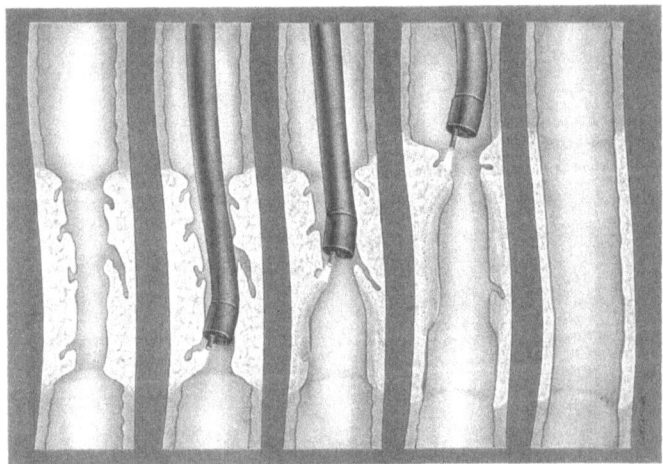

Fig. 4.5   Tumour stenosis passable to the endoscope: beginning of laser therapy working in oral direction

the circles described by the laser beam. The intention is to vaporize the tissue of the central areas and to cause white necroses towards the periphery. The procedure is repeated every other day. After this interval laser oedema and necrotic tissue disappear in most cases.

The power output selected is 90–100 watts with a pulse duration of 2 s or more at a distance of 3–10 mm. Laser coagulation beginning at the proximal end of the tumour stenosis is associated with an increased risk of perforation. The complication rate has been reported to be between 12 and 30%[34, 37, 46].

In our experience, initiating laser application at the distal end and working oral-ward is much easier, and there is less danger of perforation (Figs. 4.5, 4.6). The big advantage of this technique is that the direction of the intestinal axis is permanently visualized. Dilatation of the tumour stenosis is a necessary additional procedure prior to coagulation.

A third possibility is application of the laser along a laser-resistant guide probe as described by Ell[47] (Fig. 4.7). The guide probe is passed through the stenosis under endoscopic or fluoroscopic control. Coagulation is begun at the proximal margin of the tumour and the laser works around the laser-resistant guide probe in the distal direction, until the lumen is visualized or the stenosis can be negotiated with the endoscope. Integrated within the guide probe is an aspiration channel, through which smoke and CO_2 gas can be suctioned off.

Results Between 1 June 1984 and 31 August 1985, 62 patients with malignant stenoses of the uppergastrointestinal tract were submitted to laser therapy at the Medical Department of the University Hospital Erlangen. Twenty-three of the patients (37.1%) were curatively inoperable, 39 (62.9%) were inoperable for general reasons such as age or additional serious illness. Table 4.2 shows the location, degree and length of stenoses.

In the case of a tumour stenosis permitting passage of the endoscope, laser therapy was employed as the sole method, otherwise a combination of dilatation and laser therapy, or laser therapy along a laser-resistant guide probe, was used. On average, three laser sessions (range 2–6) and two dilatation sessions (range 1–5) proved necessary. The time interval between the treatment steps was usually 1 day.

An average of 3200 joules (range 1000–10 000) of energy were

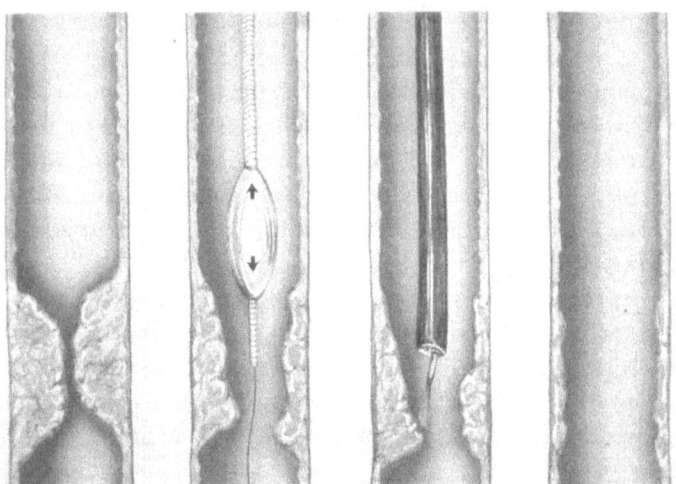

Fig. 4.6   Tumour stenosis requiring combined therapy by dilatation (Eder-Puestow dilator) and laser coagulation, working from distal to proximal margin

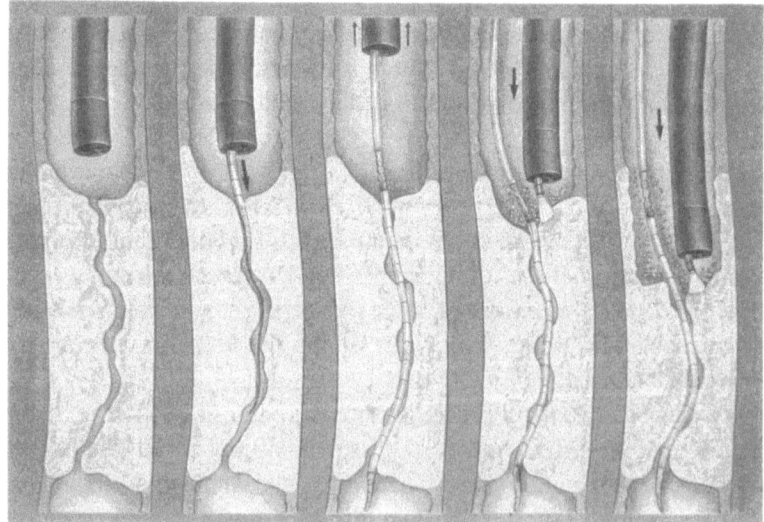

Fig. 4.7   Laser therapy carried out along the laser-resistant guide probe from proximal to distal in a filiform stenosis; the correct direction is guided by the probe

Table 4.2 Tumour characteristics prior to laser therapy ($n = 62$), Medical Department, University Hospital, Erlangen

Localization		Degree of stenosis	
Oesophagus	39	Stenosis endoscopically	37 (59.6%)
proximal	5	impassable	
middle	18	(lumen < 9 mm)	
distal	16		
Stomach (cardia)	15	length of stenosis	
Anastomosis		> 4 cm	32 (51.6%)

Table 4.3 Results of palliative laser therapy ($n = 62$), Medical Department, University Hospital, Erlangen

Initial treatment successful	50/62 patients (80.6%)
(solid food can be eaten)	
Complications (total)	3/62 patients (4.8%)
Perforation	2/62 patients
Esophago-mediastinal fistula	1/62 patients
Mortality	1/62 patients (1.6%)
Dysphagia-free interval	
3–6 weeks	29/42* patients (69.1%)
> 3 months	9/42* patients (21.4%)

* 20 patients were not followed up

employed per session. The total energy applied during initial treatment varied considerably, depending upon the tumour on the average 8900 joules (range 4800–63 000) were applied.

At the end of treatment, four-fifths of the patients were able to eat solid food again (Table 4.3). In 12 patients the objective of treatment was not achieved. Of these, three patients had stenoses with invasion of the larynx and neurological problems in swallowing. Four patients were able to take only liquids after treatment, although the endoscope could readily be passed through the extended stenosis. One patient was in an extremely debilitated condition; one patient refused further treatment after the first laser session.

In three patients (4.8%) severe complications were observed (Table 4.3). In the first case, during laser therapy the patient who had previously undergone radiotherapy revealed an oesophago-mediastinal fistula which, in the same session, was closed with a rapidly hardening amino acid solution applied via the endoscope. In a second patient perforation into the abdominal cavity occurred and required surgical repair. In the third case, after bougienage and laser therapy of a bronchial carcinoma, perforation leading to septic mediastinitis and subsequent death occurred.

In somewhat more than two-thirds of the patients who presented themselves for follow-up examination, a clinically relevant recurrent stenosis occurred after 3–6 weeks (Table 4.3). Recurrence-free intervals of more than 3 months were the exception rather than the rule.

The experience of the Erlangen Clinic was confirmed by an inquiry carried out by Ell[19] covering a total of 1359 patients (Tables 4.4–4.6).

Alternatives to laser therapy

Possible non-surgical alternatives to laser coagulation are: long-term bougienage, implantation of 'bridging' endo-prostheses; radiotherapy, including after-loading; and chemotherapy with cytotoxic agents: sclero-therapy of tumour stenoses[48], electroresection[49], 'hot bougienage'[50], percutaneous endoscopically controlled gastrostomy (PEG), or the creation of a Witzel fistula, are rarely employed.

Implantation of intestinal bridging tubes The method of implanting oesophageal endoprostheses, which is largely employed today under combined endoscopic and fluoroscopic control, has been standardized[51–57].

The indication for the implantation of an oesophageal 'bridging tube' is tumour stenosis in oesophageal, cardiac or gastric carcinoma, bronchial and mediastinal tumours, and oesophago-bronchial fistulae, usually with underlying malignancy. Prerequisites for this procedure are that surgery is not indicated, radiotherapy holds out no chance of success, the tumour is located not less than 2 cm distal to the upper oesophageal sphincter, and the patient has an expected survival time of at least 4–6 weeks and is co-operative, or can be motivated.

Results At the Medical and Surgical Department of the University Hospital at Erlangen the indication for endoscopic implantation of

Table 4.4 International inquiry: patients, prior treatment and pre-therapy tumour characteristics (hospitals with > 15 treated patients. $n = 20$)

Treated patients (total) (n)	1184 (100%)
Localization	
Oesophagus	816 (68.9%)
proximal	174 (14.7%)
middle	348 (29.4%)
distal	294 (24.8%)
Stomach	265 (22.3%)
Anastomosis	100 (8.4%)
Duodenum/Jejunum	3 (0.3%)
Degree of stenosis	
Stenosis endoscopically impassable (lumen <9 mm)	600 (55.7%)
Length of stenosis >4 cm	686 (57.9%)
Pre-treatment	
Radiotherapy	152 (12.8%)
Chemotherapy	50 (4.2%)

Table 4.5 International inquiry; premedication and technical data on laser therapy (hospitals > 15 treated patients; $n = 20$)

Premedication	
Tranquillizers + analgesics	10/20
Tranquillizers	5/20
Analgesics	1/20
Hypnotics	1/20
Tranquillizers + analgesics/anaesthetics	3/20
Laser sessions (initial treatment)	
on average 3 (2–6)	
Energy emitted	
on average 11 000 (7000–24 000) joules	
Technique employed	
Combined laser therapy (laser + bougienage) and laser therapy alone	16/20
Laser therapy alone	4/20

Table 4.6 International inquiry; results of palliative laser therapy (according to Ref. 19) ($n = 1184$)

Initial treatment successful	
(solid food can be taken)	983 (83.0%)
Complications (total)	49 (4.1%)
Perforation	25 (2.1%)
Fistulas	9 (0.8%)
Haemorrhage	8 (0.7%)
Sepsis	7 (0.6%)
Complications resulting in death	12 (1.0%)

an endoprosthesis was established in 170 patients, comprising 136 men having an average age of 63.6 and 34 women with an average age of 73.2 years. In 10.9% of the cases the condition was an oesophago-tracheal fistula resulting from such neoplasms as oesophageal or lung cancer or, in one case, underlying tuberculosis. Almost 90% of the oesophageal 'bridging tubes' were implanted for the palliation of tumour stenoses.

Of the 170 tube implantations attempted, 5.8% were unsuccessful, obstruction of the tube occurred in 3.5%, and dislodgement in 7.0%, the initial failure being eliminated endoscopically by reimplantation in 5.8%. Of the 10 perforations, five were associated with the death of the patient.

On average, patients with a 'bridging tube' survived for 8 weeks, with a maximum survival of 60 weeks. In all patients in whom endo-scopic implantation was successful, a marked improvement in dys-phagia was observed.

Compared with the surgical placement of oesophageal 'bridging tubes', endoscopic endoprosthesis implantation is associated with an appreciably lower complication rate[58].

Bridging tubes and laser coagulation in tumour stenoses of the upper gastrointestinal tract As a major alternative form of treatment of tumour stenoses of the upper gastrointestinal tract, laser coagulation vies with the placement of an oesophageal 'bridging tube'. Radio-therapy and chemotherapy are usually employed in combination with the re-establishment of luminal patency through the use of the laser, or implantation of an endoprosthesis.

Table 4.7 Tumour stenosis, upper gastrointestinal tract

	'Tubes'	versus	Laser	
⊖	Implantation of plastic material	Mode of action	Diminution of tissue	⊕
⊕	90%	Success rate	90%	⊕
⊖	2–3(5)%	Lethality	1%	⊕
⊖	Dislocation perforation	Complications	Restenosing	⊖
⊕	Occlusion possible	Fistulae	Occlusion not possible	⊖
⊖		Localization		⊕
	Not possible	Proximal	Possible	
	Not possible	Distal	Possible	
	Not possible	Total stenosis	Possible	
⊕		Costs		⊖
⊕		Hospitalization		⊖

⊕ advantage
⊖ disadvantage

For this reason we first compare the advantages and disadvantages of tube implantation and laser coagulation (Table 4.7). With either technique the patency of the oesophagus can be maintained in more than 90% of cases[27, 33–35, 41, 51–57, 59, 60]. The complication rates of the two procedures are only partially comparable, since in the case of perforation, tube implantation is at the same time the treatment of choice. Furthermore, a number of complications associated with tube implantation, for example obstruction or dislocation, can be corrected by a renewed implantation. In many respects that would be comparable to re-stenosis following laser coagulation. With respect to mortality rates, a retrospective comparison can be only approximate, but it does appear that the mortality rate associated with laser coagulation – roughly 1% – is below that observed in tube implantation – approximately 2–3% up to 5% and more.

A disadvantage of prosthetic implantation is pain or pressure necrosis caused by the tube itself. The dissolution of the tube due to material failure appears to have been largely eliminated in more recent models. Further disadvantages of the 'bridging tube' are dislocation, tumour overgrowth, or penetration. On the other hand, laser coagu-

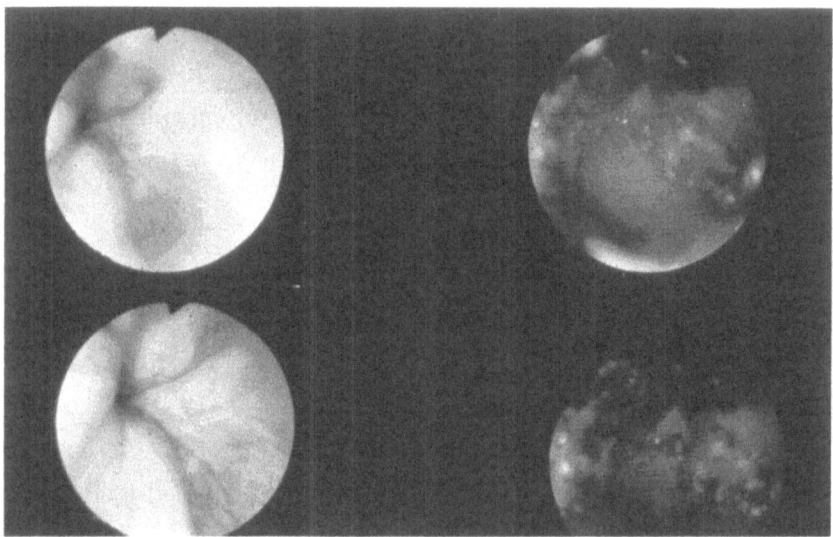

Fig. 4.8 Endoscopic aspect of tumour stenoses of the distal oesophagus before and after laser coagulation

lation offers no possibility for closing an oesophageal fistula. As a rule the opening of the tumour stenosis in the upper gastrointestinal tract by means of the laser beam requires two or three sessions; that is, a period of treatment of 1–2 weeks, while the endoprosthesis can be implanted in a single session. As a general rule laser coagulation needs to be repeated after 3–12 weeks. In addition to the cost of hospitalization, the cost of purchasing and maintaining the laser equipment must also be considered. The principal advantage of the laser is that stenosing tissue is not merely displaced, but rather that patency is re-established by the removal of tissue by vaporization, or the formation of necrosis with subsequent sloughing (Fig. 4.8). Laser coagulation is also possible in the region of the upper sphincter of the oesophagus, although considerable experience on the part of the physician is required (Figs 4.9, 4.10). In complete stenosis that cannot be negotiated even with a thin guidewire, cautious coagulation – working from the proximal margin – can initially be employed to permit the passage of the guidewire.

Before a final evaluation of the two procedures can be made a prospective study is needed, in which mortality and complication rates, time and cost factors, together with the general well-being (retrosternal pain) of the patient, are the main parameters.

When both methods are available the prosthesis will certainly be given preference in oesophago-bronchial fistulae, in the case of sub-mucous tumour growth, and also possibly in the case of long stenosis (Table 4.8). In contrast, very proximal stenosis of the oesophagus, total or bleeding stenosis with deverging axis of the oesophagus or of very firm consistency, short stenosis with the tumour involving only parts of the circumference or stenosis due to anastomotic recurrences after gastrectomy, would appear to be better dealt with by laser coagulation. This also applies to tumour stenosis associated with concomitant compression of the airways, since the introduction of an oesophageal tube can result in complete occlusion of the trachea or main bronchi.

Depending upon the experience of the endoscopist and on the facilities available, emphasis given to laser or tubes may vary. In principle it is possible to re-establish patency in a high percentage of oesophageal stenosis, through the use of bougienage, chemotherapy or radiotherapy, laser coagulation and the implantation of an endo-prosthesis. Almost any of the therapeutic procedures mentioned can be used in combination with others. In general, dilatation is employed to 'prepare the way' for tube implantation or the use of the laser. In squamous cell carcinomas, radiotherapy and chemotherapy can be combined with any other procedure, so that a total of 303 com-binations would appear possible. Finally, although the implantation of an endoprosthesis represents an alternative means for treatment of tumour stenosis in the upper digestive tract, the question 'tube or laser?' is already being answered by some authors thus: 'tube and laser'. The future will show which form of treatment or combina-tion of treatments will be given preference for the individual indica-tion.

Colorectal tumour stenoses

In comparison with stenoses of the upper gastrointestinal tract, less experience has been gained with the laser in the colorectum. However, since such non-surgical alternatives as bridging tubes or balloon dila-tation are not available, or are still being developed, there is growing

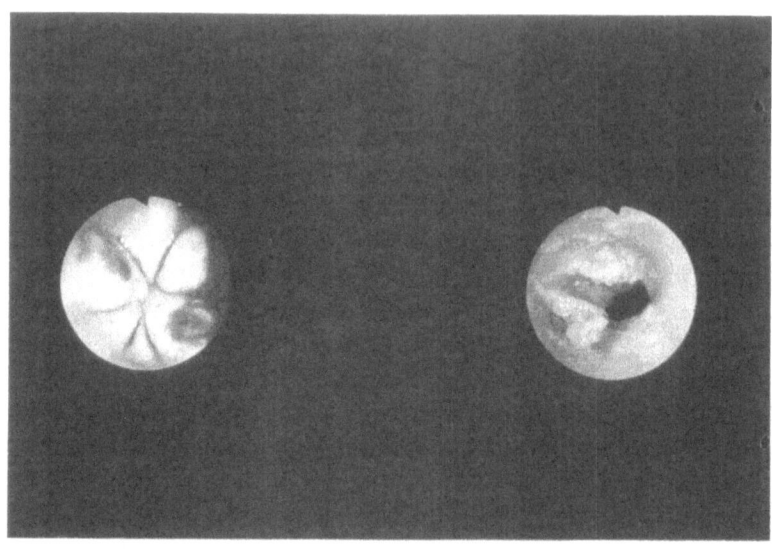

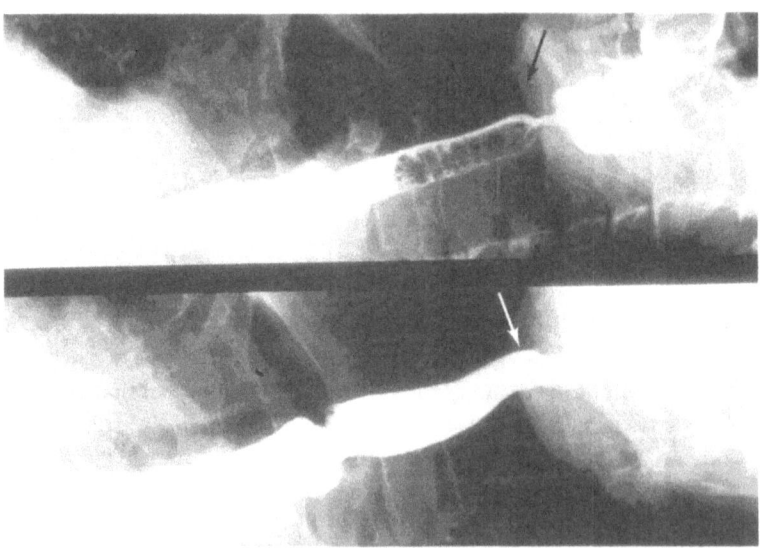

Fig. 4.9 and 10   Endoscopic and radiological aspect of a proximal tumour stenosis (↑) before and after laser therapy

Table 4.8 Tumour stenosis, upper gastrointestinal tract, therapy to be preferred

'Tubes'	*Laser*
Fistulae	Short stenosis
	'Total' stenosis
Tumour length >6 cm	Rigid stenosis, diverging axis of the
Submucosal growth	stenosis
	Proximal stenosis—tumour not
	circumferential
	Polypoid tumour
	Postoperative stenosis (oesophago-
	jejunostomy with recurrence)
	Tumour compression of respiratory tract

Table 4.9 Follow-up after palliative laser treatment of colorectal tumours[62]

Period (weeks)	*Feature of treatment*		
	Obstruction	*Bleeding*	*Obstruction +*
			bleeding
	(n = 24)	*(n = 40)*	*(n = 20)*
Deceased	8.5 (1–37)	30 (4–150)	19.5 (1–150)
Alive	52.5 (29–67)	52 (19–130)	21.5 (5–34)

interest in colorectal laser application. In contrast to the unchanging incidence of oesophageal carcinoma, colorectal carcinoma is still on the increase.

The indication for laser treatment of colorectal tumour stenosis is restricted to (1) patients who are inoperable due to widespread tumour disease (local or general metastases), or to severe secondary illness; (2) patients refusing surgical treatment; and (3) those presenting with obstruction of sudden onset in the case of left colon cancer. In our experience, laser coagulation is rarely used for haemostasis. Lambert and Sabhen[61] treated 131 patients with colorectal cancer, to the clinical benefit of most of them. Complications were rarely seen in this study. There is a large and well-documented report on laser therapy of colorectal stenoses from Amsterdam[62]. Luminal patency was reportedly restored in 20/24, and haemostasis achieved in 37/40 patients with colorectal tumour, while 19/20 patients were successfully treated for both bleeding and obstruction. Major complications were seen in 14% of the patients, and comprised perforation (six patients), stricture necessitating colostomy (three patients), and delayed post-treatment haemorrhage (two patients). The laser-related mortality rate was 3.6% (three patients). As in palliative upper GI tract tumour therapy, a wide range of treatment sessions (one to five) and applied energy (980–37 105 joules) proved necessary for effective palliation. The follow-up period varied in accordance with indication, with a longer period for those still under surveillance (Table 4.9).

Among 460 patients with colonic cancer, Kiefhaber[63] reported 57 with acute obstruction of the left colon. To avoid a two- or three-stage operation, recanalization of the stenosis was attempted to permit preoperative peroral bowel lavage and primary resection. The stenosis was successfully reopened in 54/57 patients, and two perforations were seen; there was no laser-induced mortality. Twenty-seven patients were operated on, with a mortality rate of 3.7%. Technically, laser coagulation of colonic tumours resembles that of oesophageal tumours. Coagulation is begun on the luminal side and is continued towards the site of origin of the tumour. Some authors prefer to employ pulses of 0.5–1.0 s, and a power setting of 70–100 W. CO_2 flow appears necessary to keep the fibre clean, to temporarily stop bleeding by pressure, and to avoid explosive gas mixtures. However, care must be taken to avoid over-distension of the bowel. In our experience the contact mode of laser application, and the use of a laser-resistant guide, is particularly useful in the colorectum. Results of palliative (and preoperative) laser coagulation appear encouraging – despite the fact that none of the studies reported employed an established therapy protocol, and none incorporated a control group.

Curative tumour therapy

Curative therapy of upper gastrointestinal tumours has been carried out on a large scale in the case of early carcinoma of the stomach, and also, but more rarely, in carcinoma of the oesophagus. In the colon, owing to the fact that growths are usually polypoid, polypectomy is normally the method of choice and curative laser therapy is used only exceptionally in case of villous adenomas. The use of the laser represents curative tumour therapy in case all cancer cells have been completely destroyed. This is possible only when the following conditions are met:

1. tumour invasion must not involve the full thickness of the gastrointestinal wall; and
2. regional metastases or distant metastases must be excluded.

Since, by definition, these tumours are locally operable lesions, both conditions are usually demonstrated intraoperatively by the resection of the tumour-bearing segment of the bowel and removal of the regional lymph nodes with subsequent detailed histological work-up. The pre-operative diagnostic work-up is not normally capable of showing whether the two preconditions are met. Every locally operable gastrointestinal carcinoma must be treated surgically in accordance with the requirements of cancer surgery. The sole exception is colonic carcinoma within an adenoma, when (1) the carcinoma has been removed with a margin of healthy tissue, (2) it is well or moderately well differentiated, and (3) when no spread to lymphatic or blood vessels can be demonstrated. Potentially curative laser therapy can therefore apply only to patients with locally operable carcinomas who are considered inoperable for general reasons. The establishment of general inoperability, and thus the decision to employ local laser therapy, must be documented jointly by the gastroenterologist and the surgeon.

An important diagnostic aid for establishing the depth of penetration of the tumour, is endoscopic ultrasonography[64]. The endoscopic ultrasonic picture of the wall of the stomach is characterized by five layers. Both real and virtual (border echo) layers are visualized. With the aid of comparative histological examinations, however, the echo-endoscopic layers can be correlated with the histological layers. With a certain degree of reliability the diagnosis of an early gastric carcinoma or early carcinoma of the oesophagus can therefore be confirmed by the echo-endoscopic appearance. The reservation is that the diagnosis is macroscopic and not histological. In no case can lymph node metastases of a carcinoma of the stomach be excluded on the basis of endoscopic ultrasonography. Only in the case of advanced carcinoma of the oesophagus can echo-endoscopy document regional lymph node metastases with a relatively high degree of reliability.

Early gastric carcinoma The experience of potentially curative laser treatment of gastric carcinoma is restricted to a comparatively small number of patients. The largest group of cases – from Japanese collected statistics – was reported by Takemoto[65] in 1986. Out of 785 patients with early carcinoma of the stomach, 427 were submitted to endoscopy 1 year after potentially curative laser therapy. A recurrent carcinoma was found in 80 cases (Table 4.10). A breakdown of the 47 early gastric carcinomas submitted to potentially curative laser coagulation by Takemoto *et al.*[65] revealed five recurrences among the 47 primary lesions 1–5 years after the operation (Table 4.11). Of interest is the breakdown of recurrences by size, macroscopic and histological type, and also by depth of penetration of the initial primary early gastric carcinoma (Table 4.12). Favourable conditions are, apparently, early carcinomas smaller than 2 cm and of type I, when the lesion is a well-differentiated carcinoma limited to the mucosa. In 14 patients, Takemoto *et al.*[65] carried out echo-endoscopic examinations prior to and after the laser treatment. Although, in all the cases, laser coagulation was considered to be adequate on the basis of the echo-endoscopic image, recurrent carcinoma developed in two of the 14 cases (after 22 and 10 months).

Recently, photosensitizing substances have been employed in the treatment of gastric carcinoma. Kato[45] reported on the use of an argon dye laser applied after the administration of haematoporphyrin derivatives (HpD). Here the ablating property of the laser is not employed. Rather the cell-destroying effect of photochemical reactions is utilized. Kato[45] treated 28 patients with carcinoma of the stomach including 17 cases of early carcinoma (10 type II, three IIa, three a combination of IIc and III, and two type I). Among 17 patients (18 lesions), complete remission was achieved in 10 (11 lesions). Among 13 resected carcinomas, complete remission was confirmed histologically in six. In 11 patients with advanced carcinoma, complete remission was achieved in none. Complete remission was defined as the failure to demonstrate residual tumour tissue, either endoscopically, grossly, or histologically; significant remission was defined as the destruction of 60% or more of the original tumour; partial remission

Table 4.10 Potential curative laser treatment of early gastric carcinoma (according to Ref. 65)

	Criteria		
Laser	a	b	c
Nd:YAG	308	73	299
	(22)	(73)	(80)
Argon	9	2	—
	(2)	(0)	—
Ar + HpD	1	0	4
	(1)	(0)	(1)
Ar-dye + HpD	28	2	50
	(4)	(0)	(14)
Others	1	3	5
	(0)	(0)	(3)
	347	80	358
	(29)	(9)	(98)

( ) Number of patients operated on after laser treatment
a = negative biopsy for > 1 year
b = positive biopsy after 1 year
c = pending; laser therapy < 1 year

Table 4.11 Follow-up after potential curative laser therapy of early gastric carcinoma (according to Ref. 65)

n	Follow-up (years)	Cancer in biopsy	
		Positive	Negative
1	5	—	1
11	4	1	10
6	3	—	6
14	2	3	11
15	1	1	14
47			

Table 4.12 Rate of cancer recurrences after potential curative laser therapy (according to Ref. 65)

		n	Cancer Negative (*continuously*)	Positive
Size	<2 cm	39	38 (98%)	1
	>2 cm	8	4 (50%)	4
Macroscopic type	Elevated	→15	15 (100%)	0
	Depressed	→32	27 (84%)	5
Histological type	Differentiated	→43	41 (95%)	2
	Undifferentiated	→ 4	1 (25%)	3
Depth of invasion	Mucosa	31	31 (100%)	0
	Submucosa	16	11 (69%)	5

20–60% of the original tumour; and no remission less than 20% of the primary tumour mass. According to the authors, problems continue to exist owing to the photosensitivity of the skin. Furthermore, difficulties in achieving a uniform distribution of the HpD, or in penetrating into deeper tissue layers, are still encountered. To date it would appear that successful treatment is possible only with small superficial tumours.

In the case of early carcinoma of the stomach, resection done in accordance with the requirements of cancer surgery continues to offer the best chance of achieving a cure. As experience gained to date shows, only in patients considered inoperable for general reasons is laser coagulation of the early gastric carcinoma in curative intent permitted; an echo-endoscopic surveillance is desirable. In any case, regular endoscopic and bioptic follow-up examinations must be ensured.

Benign strictures – benign tumours (precancerous lesions)

So far there are only a few anecdotal reports on the use of laser therapy to treat benign strictures[60, 66]. The best results appear to be obtained in the case of post-operative stricture. Little experience has been gained to date with the treatment of stenoses in Crohn's disease. Controlled studies comparing laser and conventional dilatation therapy are not available.

Potentially curative laser treatment of precancerous lesions has been reported in the case of gastric and colorectal adenomas[67-70].

Rösch and Frühmorgen[67] reported argon laser treatment in 3/12 patients with flat adenoma of the stomach ('borderline lesion') following snare-ectomy of the premalignant lesion. Kato[69] employed Nd:YAG laser coagulation to treat 14 broad-based 'borderline lesions' in 12 patients; no complications were observed. Post-laser ulceration healed within 4–7 weeks and afterwards no atypical epithelium was to be seen.

A decision to employ laser therapy in the treatment of precancerous lesions has, however, greater significance in the colorectum. There are also more anecdotal reports on laser ablation of colorectal polyps. The largest and best-documented study, covering 100 patients, was published by Mathus-Vliegen and Tytgat[70].

Among 26 patients with extensive adenoma growth (more than two-thirds of the circumference, or longitudinal extension more than 4 cm) complete tumour ablation was achieved in only eight, as determined by endoscopic and histological criteria. Relief of symptoms (diarrhoea, excessive mucus discharge, haematochezia, iron deficiency anaemia, faecal incontinence, hypokalaemina and dehydration) was accomplished in 15/16 patients. Follow-up over a median of 94 weeks revealed recurrence/persistence of adenomatous tissue in 18 patients; in five patients carcinoma was detected in biopsy material obtained from the ground of the laser ulcer. Major complications occurred in 11.6% of this group, stenosis in 7.7% and perforation in 3.9%.

Among 22 patients with adenomas of between 1 and 4 cm in diameter, a high percentage of symptomatic relief was achieved (13/22 patients). After a median follow-up period of 44 weeks, complete ablation was observed in 10/22 patients. Carcinoma was demonstrated in five patients; post-treatment haemorrhage occurred as a complication in 9%.

The results obtained in patients with adenomas less than 1 cm were better. Adenoma recurrence/persistence was found in 1/19 patients after an overall follow-up period of 16 weeks; no malignancy was discovered, and no major complication occurred.

In conclusion, it may be said that in adenomas more than 1 cm the symptoms were very effectively controlled, but sustained ablation of neoplastic tissue was accomplished in only a moderate 40% of the cases. Major complications occurred in about 10% of the patients; carcinoma was detected after laser therapy in 10/40 (25%) of the larger adenomas.

In a second group comprising 21 patients with familial polyposis submitted to subtotal colectomy and ileorectal anastomosis, Mathus-Vliegen and Tytgat detected no malignancy after repeated laser therapy within the rectal stump (follow-up 5 years).

In the case of precancerous lesions, laser coagulation is performed at lower energy levels, that is, 40–50 W). There has been no definitive decision on whether to use a stippling (dotted) or a sweeping, 'paint-brush' technique for laser application; the latter technique does, however, appear to induce more scarring and stenoses.

On the basis of the results presented by Mathus-Vliegen and Tytgat, it must be concluded that laser therapy of benign adenomas, in par-ticular those with a diameter over 1 cm, should be restricted to patients who are inoperable for general reasons. This will apply until certain questions have been answered; for example, how deeply the lesions must be destroyed, or how malignancy in large villous adenomas is to be detected.

A further prerequisite for laser therapy in the lesions mentioned is that close follow-up must be guaranteed both by the endoscopist and the patient.

The major drawback of laser therapy is the lack of a complete histological examination. The result is that the endoscopist is (often) not aware whether he is dealing with a benign precancerous lesion, or with a frank carcinoma. Whenever possible the aim must be a total 'biopsy' and histological work-up, whether by trans-abdominal or trans-anal surgery (method according to Buess). A further drawback of laser coagulation is that subsequent excision of the mucosal lesion is impaired by scarring. In the case of inoperable patients, laser therapy of benign precancerous lesions has produced promising results, but the persistence/recurrence rate seems to be higher (40%) than after surgery (17%)[71]. According to Tytgat[72] there is still no evidence that laser therapy of benign precancerous lesions represents progress in the case of the patient with an average surgical risk.

COAGULATIVE LASER THERAPY

Gastrointestinal bleeding

The initial application of the laser in the gastrointestinal tract was the treatment of active or potential bleeding. Goodale[80] was the first author to report on successful haemostasis with the CO_2 laser in animal experiments.

The development of laser coagulation as a technique for stopping bleeding underwent several phases. The first phase was characterized by reports on experiments carried out on animals. Here, for the most part, the argon and Nd:YAG laser were employed[73-81,83]. The second phase was characterized by case reports of laser coagulations in the gastrointestinal tract[2,82,83a]. The third phase followed with reports on larger numbers of patients in whom haemostasis by laser coagulation had proved successful[25,26,84,85]. The compilations were impressive because of the large number of patients involved, and the high rate of success achieved. In most cases no information was provided on re-bleeding rates. Since these studies were 'uncontrolled', conclusions as to the effect of laser coagulation on such prognostic factors as mortality, length of hospitalization, incidence of operation or trans-fusion rates cannot be drawn with any degree of certainty. Despite these reservations, the commercialization of laser technology for use in gastrointestinal haemostasis began in this phase. Therefore controlled studies, which were initiated in the fourth and last phase, have been carried out only to a limited extent. So far, comparative investigations have been reported only in references 86–96. With the exception of Fleischer[31], who coagulated patients with acute oesophageal variceal bleeding, most of the other studies are concerned primarily with haemorrhages from peptic lesions.

The discussion as to which laser would be best suited for haemostasis in the gastrointestinal tract arose at an early date. Since no flexible transmission system was available for the CO_2 laser, attention was concentrated on the argon and the Nd:YAG lasers. A major argument in favour of the argon laser was its maximum absorption in the red–green range. As a result of this property, the depth of penetration of this laser is smaller than that of the Nd:YAG laser. Animal exper-iments suggested that the argon laser would be associated with a lower complication rate and greater safety[73,74]. The higher energy level of

99

the Nd:YAG laser promised more effective haemostasis[37,81]. It is very likely that future discussions of this topic will include other lasers with additional properties with respect to the most commonly employed laser systems to date – the argon and Nd:YAG lasers – the following remarks can be made: both lasers can control gastrointestinal bleeding; the argon laser is possibly somewhat safer, although in controlled studies a remarkably low complication rate has also been reported for the Nd:YAG laser. As a result of the greater energy applied, the use of the Nd:YAG laser appears somewhat easier, since haemostatic effects can still be achieved from a greater distance than with the argon laser. To date, the majority of laser users have decided in favour of the Nd:YAG laser system.

Method Before attempting to accomplish endoscopic haemostasis the location and differential diagnosis of a bleeding source must be established within the framework of an emergency endoscopy. A further task of emergency endoscopy is to differentiate between an actively bleeding lesion (Forest Ia and Ib), and bleeding sources with stigmata of recent bleeding. The latter are lesions with stigmata of prior bleeding (Forrest II). Of particular importance here is the visible blood vessel, which will be discussed later. Nowadays, oesophageal varices are first treated by sclerotherapy. On account of frequent recurrent bleeding in the short term, laser coagulation has not been accepted for use in this situation.

Among almost 1500 reviewed emergency endoscopies done at the Medical Department of the University Hospital at Erlangen, combined lesions were observed in about 20% of the emergency endoscopies performed. More than two-thirds of the cases with verified sources of bleeding had peptic lesions. The distribution of potential bleeding sources roughly corresponds to that of actively bleeding sources (Table 4.13).

More than 90% of the authors employ the high-energy Nd:YAG laser. As described above, generally either a conventional fibreglass instrument (e.g. GIF Q10, Olympus) is used, or a treatment modification with a larger biopsy channel. During haemostasis a constant flow of CO_2 is recommended to cool the quartz fibre and to remove liquid blood.

Successful haemostasis by laser coagulation results in closure of the

Table 4.13 Emergency Endoscopy, Medical Department, University Hospital, Erlangen

Verified sources of bleeding (Forrest I, II) ($n = 1424$)		62.5%
Solitary	48.4%	
Multiple	14.1%	
Potential sources of bleeding (Forrest III)		26.5%
Solitary	19.0%	
Multiple	7.5%	
Undetected source of bleeding in unequivocal upper GI haemorrhage		4.0%
Normal findings		7.0%
Verified source of bleeding (Forrest I, II) ($n = 878$)		
Gastric ulcer, anastomotic ulcer		23.3%
Duodenal ulcer, duodenal erosions		22.0%
Esophageal/fundic varices		15.1%
Esophagitis		13.4%
Gastric erosions		12.8%
Mallory-Weiss syndrome and other rarer lesions		8.3%
Gastric tumours		5.1%

bleeding vessel. Application of the laser energy directly to the flowing blood results in the rapid transport of the energy – now converted into heat – away from the site of application, so that insufficient energy is available for occluding the vessel. Therefore a circular area around the bleeding vessel should first be coagulated. This way the supply of blood via the afferent limb of the vessel can be reduced, or even prevented. The subsequent coagulation of the vessel itself is usually achieved with little effort.

In our experience, the injection of adrenalin 1 : 10 000 or 1 : 100 000, as first suggested by Soehendra[98], has proved useful. With this method, Forrest Ia or Ib haemorrhages can often be arrested, which improves the preconditions for final laser coagulation.

In particular, in the presence of visible vessels, coagulation is often accompanied by an intensification of the bleeding. Not infrequently a Forrest II lesion is thereby converted into a spurting (Forrest Ia) haemorrhage. Here, too, prior injection therapy proved useful in our experience. However, to date no reports on comparative studies – including animal experiments – of laser coagulation alone, and laser coagulation after previous injection, have been published.

Results A number of uncontrolled studies[84, 85], have demonstrated that successful haemostasis can be accomplished with laser coagulation. A poll conducted by Kiefhaber revealed that, among 1729 patients, haemostasis was successfully accomplished in an average of 84% (70–100%) of the cases. No data on re-bleeding were presented. In 1982, in a total of 994 cases of acute bleeding that occurred in 625 patients from a variety of bleeding sources (ulcers, erosions, vascular anomalies, bleeding tumours, Mallory-Weiss tears, and varices), Kiefhaber[25] reported successful haemostasis in 94% of cases. Patients with chronic ulcers seemed to profit by a reduction in the lethality rate, while in the case of drug- and stress-induced ulcers the situation was less favourable. The decisive prognostic factor for the overall mortality rate was the age of the patient[98a].

One of the first controlled studies was published by Rutgeerts in 1982[94]. In an initial – admittedly uncontrolled – part of this study involving Forrest Ia bleedings (23 patients), a haemostasis rate of 87% was achieved which, however, was associated with re-bleeding in 55% of the cases. The operation rate, at 61%, was appreciably lower than that of a control group from an earlier study, namely 95%. However the mortality rate in the laser-treated group was 30%. In the second, controlled part of Rutgeerts' study (86 patients with active non-spurting bleeding), laser coagulation showed significant influence on haemostasis (100% versus 77%), on re-bleeding rate (7% versus 20%), and on the incidence rate of surgery (2% as compared with 13%). In the coagulated group the mortality rate was 13%, in the control group 15%; the difference was not statistically significant (Table 4.14). In a study by MacLeod in 1982[93], the use of the Nd:YAG laser significantly reduced the re-bleeding rate and the incidence of emergency operations. In contrast, however, the transfusion rates, the duration of hospitalization, and mortality rates were not significantly influenced by laser coagulation.

The study carried out by Swain in 1983[95] revealed a significant effect of laser coagulation on the haemostasis rate, and also on the mortality rate of the laser-treated patients, which was significantly reduced. In the studies by Ihre[88], Escourrou[86] and Kreijs[96], no significant effect of laser coagulation was determined.

In addition to the already mentioned investigations with the Nd:YAG laser, three more controlled studies with the argon laser

Table 4.14 Laser coagulation in active nonspurting gastroduodenal
bleeding (according to Ref. 97)

	Laser	Control	
No. of patients	46	40	
Bleeding stopped	46 (100%)	31 (77%)	<0.001
Bleeding recurred	3/46 (7%)	6/31 (20%)	<0.1
Operation	1 (2%)	5 (13%)	<0.1
Overall mortality	6 (13%)	6 (15%)	NS

have been published. In the trials carried out by Swain[89], out of
330 patients submitted to emergency endoscopy, 76 patients with
endoscopically observable gastroduodenal ulcers and stigmata of
recent bleeding were included in the study. Fifty-three ulcers had a
visible vessel. Eight out of 24 laser-coagulated, and 17 out of 28 control
patients experienced re-bleeding. In the control group, seven patients
died; none in the laser-coagulated group – a difference which proved
statistically significant. In a study involving 136 patients, Vallon[90] was
unable to find any significant reduction in recurrent bleeding, incidence
of surgery or mortality rate. In a small trial involving 12 patients,
Jensen[92] observed initial haemostasis in 100%; through laser coagulation, the rate of emergency operations and the rate of transfusions
were significantly reduced.

Before evaluating the results of controlled studies of photocoagulation of gastrointestinal bleeding, the prognostically important factors will be considered. Bordley[99] has once again summarized
the clinical conditions carrying an unfavourable prognosis. These
included an age of more than 75, severe secondary diseases, ascites, a
drop in blood coagulation, systemic blood pressure below 100 mmHg
(1 h after admission to hospital) and continuing haemorrhage (red
blood in the gastric tube). The fact that continuing bleeding on admission to the hospital is associated with a four to twelve times higher
mortality rate than bleeding that has stopped, was already reported
by Jones in 1956[100], Schiller in 1970[101], and Jones in 1976[102]. The large
number of variable parameters involved has so far made it impossible
for the effect of emergency endoscopy on the prognosis of patients with
gastrointestinal haemorrhage to be unequivocally demonstrated[103, 104].

The large majority of patients with gastrointestinal bleeding can expect no improvement in the prognosis from emergency endoscopy, since only about 15–25% of the patients are actively bleeding during this examination. Only 18%[105] to 48%[106] reveal a so-called visible vessel and according to these authors, have a re-bleeding rate of 56–85%. Wara[107] reported a re-bleeding rate in patients with a visible vessel of less than one-third; however, in his report further endoscopic criteria can be defined as risk factors. Additional oozing, coagula overlying the visible vessel, or location of the ulcer with 'visible' vessel in the stomach or duodenum (in contrast to a pre-pyloric ulcer). Although a number of further stigmata can be taken as signs of an increased potential recurrent bleeding, in controlled studies on laser coagulation, stratification in accordance with Forrest[108] has proved useful.

To summarize the results of the controlled trials, it is striking that perforations have apparently not occurred (in seven out of nine studies), while in the uncontrolled trials the perforation rate is 1–2%. Primary haemostasis was higher in uncontrolled studies (up to 90–100%). In some investigations laser coagulation appears to have a positive effect on haemostasis, the re-bleeding rate, transfusion rate and mortality rate. However, the improvement in the prognosis by laser coagulation of gastrointestinal haemorrhage is by no means in the range that the results of the uncontrolled studies lead us to expect. In any case, further controlled trials are necessary. It must, however, be stressed that in the (controlled) studies laser coagulation has always been compared with conservative treatment. Of importance for clinical practice, however, would be a comparison of laser coagulation with (emergency) surgery.

For clinical practice the following procedure is recommended: in the case of Forrest Ia bleeding, as a rule, immediate surgery should be the aim. Those with adequate experience with laser coagulation can attempt haemostasis, with the aim of postponing surgery to the bleeding-free interval rather than performing emergency surgery. In the case of continuing Forrest Ib bleeding, also, endoscopic haemostasis can be attempted, with its associated chances of achieving a significant improvement with respect to re-bleeding and the incidence of emergency surgery. However, a reduction in mortality has not been proved. As a rule, Forrest IIa bleeding without visible vessel should be treated conservatively: in the presence of a visible vessel, laser coagulation is associated with a significant improvement in mortality. Here, too, however, the alternative to laser therapy is surgery. Large ulcers not completely to be seen endoscopically, and ulcers located at the posterior wall of the duodenal bulb, represent the worst condition for endoscopic haemostasis. In the case of bleeding from an ulcer, a re-bleeding rate within the first 2–3 years of about 60% must be expected. For this reason, in operable patients haemostasis must always be accompanied by treatment of the ulcer disease.

Admittedly, a significant number of patients cannot be incorporated into controlled trials for ethical reasons. These are patients who cannot be referred to surgery on account of severe secondary diseases. Here, laser coagulation is promising in the treatment of acute gastrointestinal bleeding and, of course, is also justified as the only method available, although the results of controlled studies will give rise to controversial discussion.

Alternative haemostatic procedures Attempts to arrest endoscopically diagnosed bleeding with the aid of haemoclips or fast-setting resins proved to be ineffective. Alternative procedures to photocoagulation are electrocoagulation and the injection of various substances.

Electrocoagulation has the advantage that the equipment employed is transportable, i.e. mobile, and the costs compared to laser coagulation are considerably lower. In 1981 Papp[109] reported an 88% success rate for haemostasis with monopolar electro-coagulation. The study was, however, uncontrolled, and such sources of bleeding as Mallory–Weiss tears and gastritis had been included. In another uncontrolled trial on the use of bipolar electrocoagulation, Donahoe[110] achieved initial haemostasis in 11 out of 14 patients, two of whom, however, experienced recurrent bleeding within 48 h. In 1984, Kernohan[111], also using bipolar electrocoagulation, was unable to report any reduction in recurrent bleeding, transfusion rate or incidence of surgery. According to Matek[112], in uncontrolled trials, haemostasis achieved with electro-hydrothermal coagulation was comparable to that accomplished with laser coagulation.

With the injection of adrenalin at concentrations of 1:10 000 or, in our own experience, 1:100 000, or of polidocanol[98] haemostasis, comparable to that produced with laser coagulation, can be achieved. The alternative procedures listed here have the advantage of lower

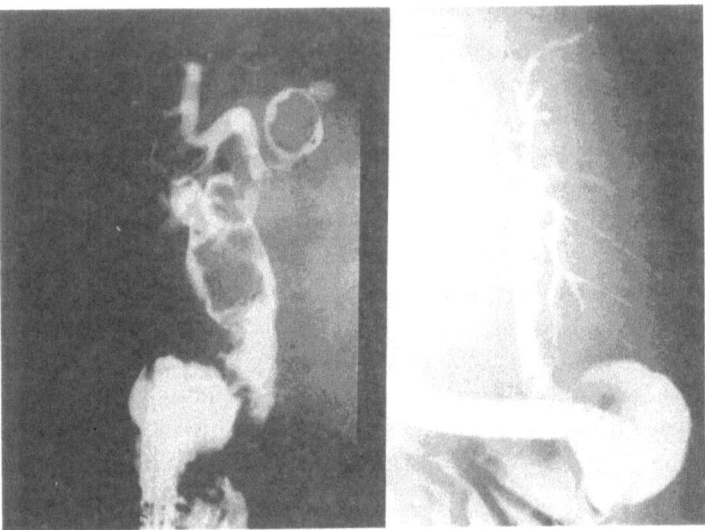

Fig. 4.11 Giant common bile duct concrement after choledochoduodenostomy before and after laser lithotripsy under visual control

cost and greater mobility. Although, on the basis of clinical experience,
they appear to be equally as successful as the laser technique, their
effectiveness has yet to be proven in controlled trials. The same applies
to the heater probe developed in recent years[113].

GALL STONE LITHOTRIPSY

In 1983 Orii *et al.*[114] reported the first successful destruction of common
bile duct stones with the aid of the Nd:YAG continuous-wave laser
in man using transcutaneous–transhepatic cholangioscopy. Later
Kouzu[115] pointed out that contact laser lithotripsy with sapphire tips
was particularly suitable for the destruction of cholesterol stones.
Mills and co-workers[116] reported *in vitro* experiments of gall stone
lithotripsy. As far as our own experiments are regarded the continuous-wave Nd:YAG laser seems ineffective for lithotripsy of gall
stones. Only thermal melting and 'drilling' effects, but no fragmentation, could be observed.

 With the aid of a flashlamp-pulsed Nd:YAG laser we
succeeded[117, 118], for the first time, in reliably and reproducibly destroy-

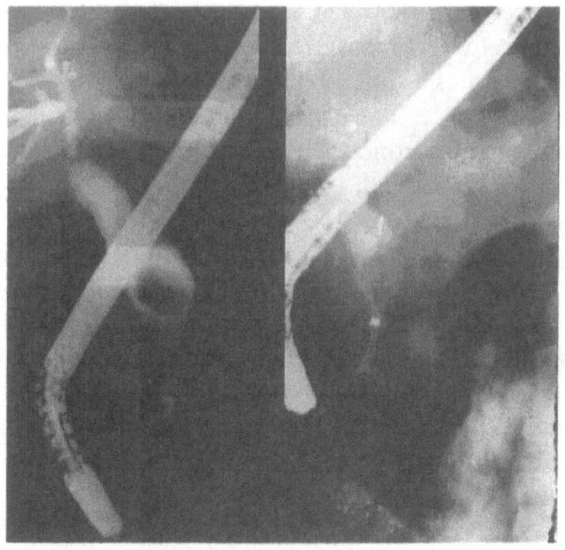

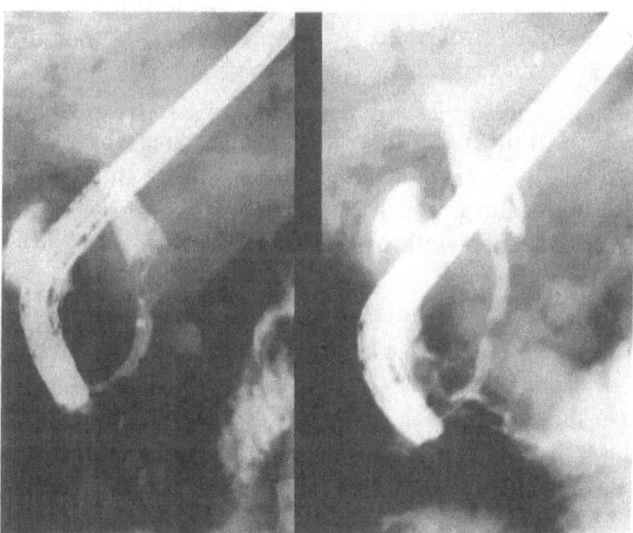

Fig. 4.12a-d Common bile duct concrement, distal narrowing of the common bile duct (**12a**); Dormia basket grasping the concrement (**12b**), lithotripsy splitting the concrements in two parts (**12c**) and concrement-free c.d. (**12d**)

ing gall stones. After *in vitro* tests animal experiments were performed. The energy required for fragmentation was between 10 and 200 joules, the pulse duration in the millisecond range, and the pulse energy between 0.15 and 2 joules. The time required to fragment the stones varied between 2 and 60 seconds. The lithotriptic effect is of a thermal nature and can be explained by the high vaporization pressures produced within the stone.

The laser light is transmitted via highly flexible glass fibre with a diameter of 0.2 mm without appreciable transmission losses, even when the fibre is strongly flexed. This was one prerequisite for endoscopic retrograde contact laser lithotripsy via conventional duodenoscopes or choledochoscopes (mother-and-baby scope).

Similar thermal lithotripsy effects can be achieved with a flashlamp-pulsed dye laser[119]. With this system, however, higher energy densities have to be applied.

Initial attempts to accomplish lithotripsy of gall stones with the aid of the Q-switched Nd:YAG laser failed due to the impossibility of coupling high pulse energies with a flexible glass fibre[120]. The use of smaller pulse energies proved to be more effective, but the attempts to break down stones regularly resulted in the destruction of the necessary opto-mechanical coupling system located at the distal tip of the light guide[121]. In the meantime we have succeeded in coupling high pulse energies of up to 50 mJ at pulse times in the nanosecond range, with a flexible glass fibre, and have been able to destroy gall stones reliably and reproducibly without any damage occurring to the distal focusing facility.

The advantage of the Q-switched laser system over the flashlamp-pulsed Nd:YAG laser is that thermal injuries to the bile duct need not be feared.

Recently we succeeded for the first time in accomplishing endoscopic retrograde laser lithotripsy of giant bile duct concrement (Figs. 4.11 and 4.12), using a pulsed Nd:YAG laser[122]. To ensure a safe distance of the quartz fibre tip from the wall of the common bile duct, various techniques, involving the use of a Dormia basket, a balloon catheter, or direct visual endoscopic control (Fig. 4.13), have been developed.

At the present time it is not possible to predict which laser system will prove useful in practical application. It is, however, to be expected that laser lithotripsy will become a preferred complementary pro-

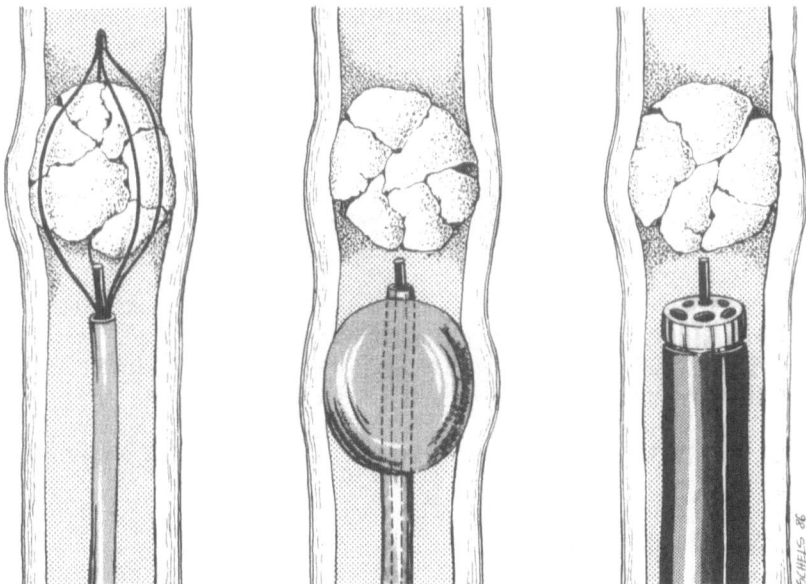

Fig. 4.13 Laser-lithotripsy by aid of (1) a Dormia basket with central laser-fibre (left); (2) a balloon catheter to avoid tissue contact of the laser fibre (middle) and (3) direct endoscopic control (right)

cedure to endoscopic papillotomy in the treatment of large common bile duct stones.

References

1. Maiman, T. H. (1960). Stimulated optical radiation in ruby lasers. *Nature*, **187**, 493
2. Frühmorgen, P., Bodem, F., Reidenbach, H. D., Kaduk, B., Demling L. and Brand, H. (1975). The first endoscopic laser coagulation in the human GI tract. *Endoscopy*, **7**, 156
3. Beesley, M. J. (1972). *Lasers and Their Applications.* (London: Taylor & Francis)
4. Svelto, O. (1982). *Principles of Lasers.* (New York: Plenum)
5. Wolbarsht, H. (1971). *Laser Applications in Medicine and Biology.* (New York: Plenum)
6. Yariv, A. (1975). *Quantum Electronics.* (New York: Wiley)
7. Boulnois, J.-L. (1986). Photophysical processes in recent medical laser developments: a review. *Lasers Med. Sci.*, **1**, 47
8. Frank, F. (1986). Technical requisites and safety considerations for the

use of the Nd:YAG lasers in gastroenterology. *Endoscopy*, **18**, 6 (Suppl. 1)

9. Meesters, E., Mester, A. F. and Mester, A. (1985). The biomedical effects of laser application. *Laser Surg. Med.*, **5**, 31
10. Dougherty, T. J. (1984). Photodynamic therapy of solid tumors. Seventy-fifth annual meeting of the American Association for Cancer Research, 9–12 May. *Proceedings*, Toronto, Canada, Vol. 25, p. 408
11. Fradin, D. W., Bloembergen, N. and Letellier, J. P. (1973). Dependence of laser-induced breakdown field strength on plasma duration. *Appl. Phys. Lett.*, **22**, 635
12. Trokel, S. L., Svinivasan, R. and Braren, B. (1983). Excimer laser surgery of the cornea. *J. Ophthalmol.*, **96**, 710
13. Berns, M. W. and Gaster, R. N. (1985). Corneal incisions produced with the 4th harmonic (266 nm) of the Nd:YAG laser. *Lasers Surg. Med.*, **5**, 371
14. Bass, M. (1986). Laser for use in medicine. *Endoscopy*, **18**, 2–5 (Suppl. 1)
15. Hofstetter, A. and Frank, F. (1979). *Der Neodym-YAG Laser in der Urologie*. Editiones Roche, p. 23
16. Hayata, Y., Kato, H., and Konaka, C. (1982). Hematoporphyrin derivative and laser photoradiation in the treatment of lung cancer. *Chest*, **81**, 269
17. Shou-Zhong Song, Jun-Heng Li, Jin Zou, Ming-Yan Shu, Fu-Yun Zhao, Mao-Lin Jin and Zhong-He Guo (1985). Hematoporphyrin derivate and laser photodynamical reaction in the diagnosis and treatment of malignant tumors. *Laser Surg. Med.*, **5**, 61
18. Nath, G. and Fidler, J. (1973). High power Nd:YAG laser surgery with a fiber-optic delivery system. *1st European Electro Optics Markets and Technology Conference, Geneva, 1972*. (Richmond: IPC Science and Technology Press, Kingprint)
19. Ell, Ch., Hochberger, J. and Lux, G. (1986). Contact and non-contact Nd:YAG laser therapy in inoperable tumour stenoses of the oesophagus and stomach – clinical experience and results. *Laser Med. Sci.*, **1**, 143
20. Sabben, G., Lambert, R. and Lenz, P. (1983). Laser therapy with quartz fibres in tissue contact. *Gastrointest. Endosc.*, **29**, 183
21. Kiefhaber, P. Moritz, K. Diagnostische und therapeutische Möglichkeiten der Endoskopie bei Polypen und Tumoren des Kolon und Rektums. Gastroent. Reihe, Hannover, 1978
22. Kiefhaber, P. (1980). *Endoscopic laser applications in gastrointestinal tract*. Proceedings of Third Asian–Pacific Congress on Digestive Endoscopy
23. Kiefhaber, P. and Kiefhaber, K. (1981). Therapeutic Nd:YAG laser application in the gastrointestial tract. In von Maercke, Y. M. F. *et al.* (eds), *Stomach Diseases – Current Status*. (Amsterdam, Oxford, Princetown: Excerpta Medica)

24. Minton, J. P. and Ketcham, A. S. (1964). The laser, a unique oncolytic entity. *Am. J. Surg.,* **108,** 845
25. Kiefhaber, P. (1982). *Laser Endoscopic Experience.* Brussels: Vth International Symposium on Digestive Endoscopy
26. Kiefhaber, P. and Kiefhaber, K. (1983). Present endoscopic laser therapy in the gastrointestinal tract. in Atsumi, K. (ed.) *New Frontiers in Laser Medicine and Surgery.* (Amsterdam, Oxford, Princetown: Excerpta Medica)
27. Kiefhaber, P. (1984). Indikationen für die endoskopische Verwendung des Lasers im Gastrointestinaltrakt. *Münch. Med. Wochemschr.,* **126,** 103
28. Kiefhaber, P., Kiefhaber, K., Huber, F. and Nath, G. (1984). Neodymium-YAG-laser application for stenosing carcinomas and neoplastic sessil polyps of the gastrointestinal tract. In Waidelich, W. *Optoelectronics in Medicine.* (Berlin, Heidelberg, New York, Tokyo: Springer)
29. Fleischer, D. E. (1982). The current status of gastrointestinal laser activity in the United States. *Gastroint. Endosc.,* **28,** 157
30. Fleischer, D. E., Kessler, F. and Hage, O. (1982). Endoscopic Nd:YAG laser therapy for carcinoma of the esophagus: a new palliative approach. *Am. J. Surg.,* **143,** 280
31. Fleischer, D. E. and Kessler, F. (1983). Endoscopic Nd:YAG laser therapy for carcinoma of the esophagus: a new form of palliative treatment. *Gastroenterology,* **85,** 600
32. Fleischer, D. E. and Sivak, M. (1983). Endoscopic Nd:YAG laser palliation for obstructing esophagogastric carcinoma. *Lasers Surg. Med.,* **3,** 172
33. Fleischer, D. E. (1984). Lasers and gastroenterology. *Gastroenterology,* **79,** 406
34. Fleischer, D. E. (1984). Endoscopic laser therapy for gastrointestinal disease. *Arch. Intern. Med.,* **144,** 1225
35. Fleischer, D. E. and Sivak, M. V. (1984). Endoscopic Nd:YAG laser therapy as palliative treatment for advanced adenocarcinoma of the gastric cardia. *Gastroenterology,* **87,** 815
36. Mellow, M., Pinkus, H., Frank, J. *et al.* (1983). Endoscopic therapy for esophageal carcinoma with Nd:YAG laser: prospective evaluation of efficacy, complications and survival. *Gastrointest. Endosc.,* **29,** 165
37. Mosquet, L. and Brunetaud, J. M. (1984). Les lasers en gastroentérologie: faut-ils s'equiper et lequel choisir. *Gastroent. Clin. Biol.,* **8,** 138
38. Riemann, J. F., Ell, Ch., Lux, G. and Demling, L. (1985). Combined therapy of malignant stenoses of the upper gastrointestinal tract by means of laser beam and bougienage. *Endoscopy,* **17,** 43
39. Ell, Ch., Riemann, J. F., Lux, G. and Demling, L. (1986). Palliative

laser treatment of malignant stenoses in the upper gastrointestinal tract. *Endoscopy*, **18**, 21 (Suppl. 1)

40. Bown, S. G., Swain, C. P., Edwards, D. A. and Salmon, P. R. (1982). Palliative relief of malignant upper gastrointestinal obstruction by endoscopic laser therapy. *Gut*, **23**, 918
41. Buset, M., Dunham, F., Baize, M., de Toeuf, J. and Cremer, M. (1983). Nd:YAG laser, a new palliative alternative in the management of esophageal cancer. *Endoscopy*, **15**, 353
42. Earlam, R. and Cunha-Melo, U. R. (1980). Oesophageal squamous cell carcinoma. *Br. J. Surg.*, **67**, 391
43. Brunetaud, J. M., Houche, P., Delmotte, J. S. *et al.* (1981). Laser in digestive endoscopy. In Atsumi and Mimsakul (eds), *Laser Tokyo 1981*. Intergroup Corp.
44. Swain, C. P., Bown, S. G. and Edwards, J. (1981). Neoplastic gastric outflow tract obstruction relieved by argon laser at endoscopy. In Atsumi and Mimsakul (eds). *Laser Tokyo 1981*. (Intergroup Corp.)
45. Kato, H., Kawaguchi, M., Konaka, C., Nishimiya, K. Kawate, N., Yoneyams, K., Kinoshita, K., Noguchi, M., Ishii, M., Shirai, M., Hirano, T., Aizawa, K. and Hayata, Y. (1986). Evaluation of photodynamic therapy in gastric cancer. *Lasers Med. Sci.*, **1**, 67
46. Delvaux, J. and Escourrou, J. (1985). Complications observées au cours du traitment par laser des tumeurs du tractus digestif supérieur. *Acta Endosc.*, **15**, 13
47. Ell, Ch., Hochberger, J., Riemann, J. F., Lux, G. and Demling, L. (1986). Laser guide for laser treatment of malignant stenoses. *Endoscopy*, **18**, 27
48. Soehendra, N., Grimm, H. and Schreiber, H. W. (1984). Endoskopische Injektionsbehandlung bei benignen und malignen Ösophagustumoren. *Deutsch. Med. Wochenschr.*, **109**, 1973
49. Classen, M. and Stock, M. (1979). Palliative tumour therapy: endoscopic tumour resection and incision: In Demling, L. and Koch, H. (eds), *Operative Endoscopy*. (Stuttgart, New York: Schattauer)
50. Kessler, B., Wittrin, G., Arndt, M. and Kohaus, H. (1981). Thermobougierung als Alternative in der Behandlung des inoperablen stenosierenden Ösophaguskarzinoms. In Häring, R. (ed.), *Chirurgie des Ösophaguskarzinoms*. (Basel: Edition Medizin, Weinheim, Deerfield)
51. Tytgat, G. N., den Hartog Jager, F. C. A. and Haverkamp, H.-J. (1976). Positioning of a plastic prosthesis under fiberendoscopic control in the palliative treatment of cardioesophageal cancer. *Endoscopy*, **8**, 180
52. Tytgat, G. N. and den Hartog Jager, F. C. A. (1977). Non-surgical treatment of cardio esophageal obstruction – role of endoscopy. *Endoscopy*, **9**, 211
53. Tytgat, G. N. (1980). Endoscopic methods of treatment of gastrointestinal and biliary stenosis. *Endoscopy*, **12**, 57 (Suppl.)

54. Tytgat, G. N. and den Hartog Jager, F. C. A. (1982). Ergebnisse der endoskopischen Implantation von Überbrückungstuben. *Dtsch. Ärzteblatt*, **79**, 49
55. Den Hartog Jager, F. C. A., Bartelman, J. F. W. M. and Tytgat, G. N. (1979). Palliative treatment of obstructing esophagogastric malignancy by endoscopic positioning of a plastic prosthesis. *Gastroenterology*, **77**, 1008
56. Lux, G., Groitl, H., Riemann, J. F. and Demling, L. (1983). Tumor stenosis of the upper gastrointestinal tract – non-surgical therapy by bridging tubes. *Endoscopy*, **15**, 207 (Suppl.)
57. Lux, G., Groitl, H. and Ell, Ch. (1986). Tumor stenoses of the upper gastrointestinal tract – therapeutic alternatives to laser therapy. *Endoscopy*, **18**, 37, (Suppl. 1)
58. Lishman, A. H., Dellipiani, A. W. and Devlin, H. B. (1980). The insertion of oesophagogastric tubes in malignant oesophageal strictures: endoscopy of surgery. *Br. J. Surg.*, **67**, 257
59. Sander, R., Poesl, H. and Spuhler, A. (1986). Therapie gastrointestinaler Tumoren mit Laser. *Internist*, **26**, 22
60. Sander, R. and Poesl, H. (1986). Treatment of non-neoplastic stenoses with the neodymium–YAG laser. *Endoscopy*, **18**, 53 (Suppl. 1)
61. Lambert, R. and Sabben, G. (1983). Laser therapy for colorectal neoplasms. *Laser Surg. Med.*, **3**, 147
62. Mathus-Vliegen, E. M. H. and Tytgat, G. N. J. (1986). Nd:YAG–laser photocoagulation in gastroenterology: its role in palliation of colorectal cancer. *Lasers Med. Sci.*, **1**, 75
63. Kiefhaber, P., Kiefhaber, K. and Huber, F. (1986). Preoperative neodymium–YAG laser treatment of obstructive colon cancer. *Endoscopy*, **18**, 44 (Suppl. 1)
64. Heyder, N., Lux, G., Riemann, J. F. and Lutz, H. (1986). Ultraschallendoskopie. *Dtsch. Med. Wochenschr.*, **111**, 324
65. Takemoto, T. (1986). Laser therapy of early gastric carcinoma. *Endoscopy*, **18**, 32 (Suppl. 1)
66. Löffler, A., Dienst, C. and Velasco, S. B. (1986). International survey of laser therapy in benign gastrointestinal tumors and stenoses. *Endoscopy*, **18**, 62 (Suppl. 1)
67. Rösch, W. and Frühmorgen, P. (1980). Endoscopic treatment of precancerosis and early gastric carcinoma. *Endoscopy*, **12**, 109
68. Richey, G. D. and Dixon, J. A. (1981). Ablation of atypical gastric mucosa and recurrent polyps by endoscopic application of lasers. *Gastrointest. Endosc.*, **27**, 224
69. Kato, O., Hattori, K., Suzuki, T., Mishio, K. and Shimizu, Y. (1984). Endoscopic Nd:YAG laser therapy for gastro borderline lesions *Gastrointest. Endosc.*, **30**, 77
70. Mathus-Vliegen, E. M. H. and Tytgat, G. N. T. (1986). Nd:YAG laser

photocoagulation in colorectal adenoma. Evaluation of its safety, usefulness, and efficacy. *Gastroenterology*, **90**, 1865

70a. Buess, G., Theiss, R. and Hütterer, F. (1984). Endoskopische Operationen in der Rektumhöhle. In *Endoskopische Techniken*. (Koln: Deutsch. Arzte Verlag)

71. Häring, R., Karavias, T. and Konradt, J. (1978). Die posteriore Proctorectomie. *Chirurg.*, **99**, 337

72. Tytgat, G. N. (1986). Benign stenosis, benign tumors. *Endoscopy*, **18**, (Suppl. 1), 60

73. Frühmorgen, P., Reidenbach, H. D. and Bodem, F. (1974). Experimental examinations on laser endoscopy. *Endoscopy*, **6**, 116

74. Frühmorgen, P., Kaduk, B., Reidenbach, H. D., Bodem, F., Demling, L. and Brand, H. (1975). Long term observations in endoscopic laser coagulations in the gastrointestinal tract. *Endoscopy*, **7**, 189

75. Katon, R. M. (1976). Experimental control of gastrointestinal hemorrhage via the endoscope: a new era dawns. *Gastroenterology*, **70**, 7

76. Protell, R. L., Silverstein, F. E., Piercey, J. *et al.* (1976). A reproducible animal model of acute bleeding ulcer – the 'ulcer marker'. *Gastroenterology*, **71**, 4

77. Silverstein, F. E., Auth, D. C., Rubin, C. E. *et al.* (1976). High power argon laser treatment via standard endoscopes. *Gastroenterology*, **71**, 558

78. Silverstein, F. E., Protell, R. L., Piercey, J. *et al.* (1977). Comparison of the efficacy of high and low power photocoagulation in control of severely bleeding experimental ulcers in dogs. *Gastroenterology*, **71**, 481

79. Silverstein, F. E., Protell, R. L., Gilbert, D. A. *et al.* (1979). Argon vs. neodymium YAG laser photocoagulation of experimental canine gastric ulcers. *Gastroenterology*, **77**, 491

80. Goodale, R., Okada, A. and Gonzales, R. (1970). Rapid endoscopic control of bleeding gastric erosions by laser radiation. *Arch. Surg.*, **101**, 211

80a. Bown, S. G., Salmon, P. R., Storey, D. W. *et al.* (1980). Nd:YAG laser photocoagulation in the dog stomach. *Gut*, **21**, 818

81. Kiefhaber, P., Nath, G., Moritz, K., Gorisch, W., Kreitmaier, A., Schramm, W. (1976). Eigenschaften verschiedener Lasertransmissionssysteme und ihre Eignung für die endoskopische Blutstillung. In Lindner, H. (ed) *Fortschritte der gastroenterologischen Endoskopie*, vol. 7, p. 144 (Baden-Baden: Witzstrock)

82. Dwyer, R., Yellin, A. and Craig, J. (1976). Gastric hemostasis by laser phototherapy in man. *J. Am. Med. Assoc.*, **23**, 1383

83. Geboes, K., Rutgeerts, P., Vantrappen, G. *et al.* (1980). A microscopic and ultrastructural study of hemostasis after laser photocoagulation. *Gastrointest. Endosc.*, **26**, 131

83a. Kiefhaber, P., Nath, G. and Moritz, K. (1977). Endoscopical control of massive gastrointestinal haemorrhage by irradiation with a high-power neodymium YAG laser. *Prog. Surg.*, **15**, 140

84. Kiefhaber, P., Moritz, K., Schildberg, F. W. *et al.* (1978). Endoskopische Nd:YAG-Laserkoagulation blutender akuter und chronischer Ulzera. *Langenbecks Arch. Chir.*, 567

85. Kiefhaber, P. (1979). *International experience with lasers for gastrointestinal bleeding.* Detroit: Proceedings of International Laser Congress

86. Escourrou, J. (1981). Nd:YAG laser therapy for acute gastrointestinal hemorrhage. In Atsumi, and Mimsakul, (eds) *Laser Tokyo 1981.* (Intergroup Corp.)

87. Rohde, H., Thorr, K., Fischer, M. *et al.* (1980). Early endoscopy combined with endoscopic neodymium YAG laser therapy in patients with actively bleeding lesions. *Abstracts of the IV European Congress of GI Endoscopy, E.,* **30.3**, 107

88. Ihre, T., Johansson, C., Seligsson, U. *et al.* (1981). Endoscopic YAG laser treatment in massive UGI bleeding. *Scand. J. Gastroenterol.,* **16**, 633

89. Swain, C. P., Storey, D. W., Northfield, T. C. *et al.* (1981). Controlled trial of argon laser photocoagulation in bleeding peptic ulcers. *Lancet,* **2**, 1313

90. Vallon, A. G., Cotton, P. B., Laurence, B. M. *et al.* (1981). Randomized trial of endoscopic laser photocoagulation in bleeding peptic ulcers. *Gut,* **22**, 228

91. Fleischer, D. E. (1982). Nd:YAG laser therapy for active variceal bleeding. *Gastroenterology,* **82**, 1058

92. Jensen, D. M., Machicado, G. A., Tapia, J. F. *et al.* (1982). Endoscopic argon laser photocoagulation of patients with severe gastrointestinal bleeding. *Gastrointest. Endosc.,* **28**, 151

93. MacLeod, I., Mills, P. R. and MacKenzie, J. F. (1982). Nd:YAG laser photocoagulation for major acute upper gastrointestinal haemorrhage. *Gut,* **23**, 905

94. Rutgeerts, P., Vantrappen, G., Broebaert, L., Janssens, J., Coremans, G., Geboes, K. and Schurmans, P. (1982). Controlled trial of YAG laser treatment of upper digestive hemorrhage. *Gastroenterology,* **83**, 410

95. Swain, C. P., Bown, S. G. and Salmon, P. (1983). Controlled trial of Nd:YAG laser photocoagulation in bleeding peptic ulcers. *Lasers Surg. Med.,* **3**, 111

96. Kreijs, G. J., Little, K. H., Westergaard, H., Hamilton, J. K. and Polter, D. E. (1985). Laser photocoagulation for the treatment of acute peptic ulcer bleeding. *Gastroenterology,* **88**, 1457 (abstract)

97. Rutgeerts, P., Vantrappen, G., Geboes, K. *et al.* (1981). Safety and efficacy of neodymium-YAG laser photocoagulation: an experimental study in dogs. *Gut,* **22**, 38

98. Soehendra, N., Grimm, H. and Stenzel, M. (1985). Injection of non-variceal bleeding lesions of the upper gastrointestinal tract. *Endoscopy*, **17**, 129

98a. Feifel, G., Letzel, H. and Heberer, G. (1979). Chirurgische Blutstillung im Zeitalter des Lasers. In Demling, L. and Rösch, W. (eds). *Operative Endoskopy*. (Berlin: Acron)

99. Bordley, D. R., Mushlin, A. I., Dolan, J. G., Richardson, W. S., Barry, M., Polis, J. and Griner, P. F. (1985). Early clinical signs identify lower-risk patients with acute upper gastrointestinal hemorrhage. *J. Am. Med. Assoc.*, **253**, 3282

100. Jones, F. A. (1956). Haematemesis – and melaena. *Gastroenterology*, **30**, 166

101. Schiller, K. R. F., Truelove, S. C. and Williams, D. G. (1970). Haematemesis and melaena with special references to factors influencing the outcome. *Br. Med. J.*, **2**, 7

102. Jones, P. F., Johnston, S. J., McEwand, A. S., Kyle, J. and Needham, L. D. (1976). Further haemorrhage after admission to hospital for gastrointestinal haemorrhage. *Br. Med. J.*, **2**, 660

103. Conn, H. O. (1981). To scope or not to scope. *N. Engl. J. Med.*, **304**, 967

104. Eastwood, G. L. (1981). Does the patient with upper gastrointestinal bleeding benefit from endoscopy? Reflections and discussion of recent literature. *Dig. Dis. Sci.*, **26**, 225

105. Griffith, W. J., Neumann, D. A. and Welsh, J. D. (1979). The visible vessel as an indicator of uncontrolled or recurrent gastrointestinal hemorrhage. *N. Engl. J. Med.*, **300**, 1411

106. Storey, D. W., Bown, S. G., Swain, C. P., Salmon, P. R., Kirkham, J. S. and Northfield, T. C. (1981). Endoscopic prediction of recurrent bleeding in peptic ulcers. *N. Engl. J. Med.*, **305**, 915

107. Wara, P. (1985). Endoscopic prediction of major rebleeding – a prospective study of stigmata of hemorrhage in bleeding ulcer. *Gastroenterology*, **88**, 1209

108. Forrest, J. A. H., Finlayson, N. D. C. and Shearman, D. J. C. (1974). Endoscopy in gastrointestinal bleeding. *Lancet*, **2**, 394

109. Papp, J. P. (1981). Electrocoagulation in upper gastrointestinal bleeding. *Dig. Dis. Sci.*, **26**, 413

110. Donahoe, P. E., Mobarhan, S., Layden, T. J. and Nyhus, L. M. (1984). Endoscopic control of upper gastrointestinal hemorrhage with a bipolar coagulation device. *Surg. Gynecol. Obstet.*, **159**, 113

111. Kernohan, R. M., Anderson, J. R., McKelvey, S. T. D. and Kennedy, T. L. (1984). A controlled trial of bipolar electrocoagulation in patients with upper gastrointestinal bleeding. *Br. J. Surg.*, **71**, 889

112. Matek, W. and Demling, L. (1986). Hemostasis – therapeutic alternatives to the laser. *Endoscopy*, **18**, 17 (Suppl. 1)

113. Auth, D. C. (1985). Endoscopic heater probe coagulation. *Gastrointest. Endosc.*, **31**, 135
114. Orii, K., Ozaki, A., Takase, Y. and Iwasaki, Y. (1983). Lithotomy of intrahepatic and choledochal stones with YAG-laser. *Surg. Gynecol. Obstet.*, **156**, 485
115. Kouzu, T., Yamazaki, Y., Maruyama, M. and Murashima, M. (1985). Cholangioscopic lithotomy using Nd-YAG laser by means of contact-type rod. 2nd Nd:YAG laser conference, München 1985
116. Mills, T. N., Watson, G. N., Swain, C. P., Bown, S. G., Wickham, J., Salmon, P. R. and Clifton, J. S. (1983). Thermal vs. photoacoustic fragmentation of urinary and biliary calculi using continuous wave and giant pulse lasers. *Laser Surg. Med.*, **3**, 156
117. Ell, Ch., Hochberger, J., Müller, D., Zirngibl, H., Giedl, J., Lux, G. and Demling, L. (1986). Laser lithotripsy of gallstone by means of a pulsed neodymium–YAG laser – *in vitro* and animal experiments. *Endoscopy*, **18**, 92
118. Ell, Ch., Wondrazek, F., Frank, F., Hochberger, J., Lux, G. and Demling, L. (1986). Laser-induced shockwave lithotripsy of gallstones. *Endoscopy*, **18**, 95
119. Watson, G. M., Jacques, S. L., Dretler, S. P. and Parrish, J. A. (1985). Tunable pulsed dye laser for fragmentation of biliary calculi. *Lasers Surg. Med.*, **5**, 189
120. Bown, S. G., Mills, T. N., Watson, G. N., Swain, C. P., Wickham, J. E. and Salmon, P. R. (1984). Laser fragmentation of biliary calculi. XII. International Congress of Gastroenterology, Lisboa, Portugal, 16–22 September
121. Hofmann, R. and Schütz, W. (1984). Zerstörung von Harnsteinen durch Laserstrahlung. Experimentelle Grundlagen und *in vitro*-Versuche. *Urologe A*, **23**, 181
122. Lux, G., Ell, Ch., Hochberger, J., Müller, D. and Demling, L. (1986). The first successful endoscopic retrograde laser lithotripsy of common bile duct stones in man using a pulsed neodymium YAG laser. *Endoscopy*, **18**
123. Laurence, B. H., Vallon, A. G., Cotton, P. B., *et al.* (1980). Endoscopic laser photocoagulation for bleeding peptic ulcers. *Lancet*, **1**, 124

5

Endoscopic Sonography of the Upper Gastrointestinal Tract: the Present Position

H. Dancygier and M. Classen

The development of morphologically oriented methods has considerably increased our diagnostic capabilities. Sonography plays a leading role in the diagnosis of hepatobiliary, pancreatic and gastrointestinal diseases. It may be used for screening purposes as well as in frequent follow-up investigations. Despite this progress there still remain regions that cannot be accurately depicted even with the most sophisticated imaging modalities presently available. The wall of the gastrointestinal tract and its immediate surroundings may be seen on computed tomographic scanning and with conventional ultrasound, but the systematic and detailed examination of these structures with transcutaneous ultrasonography and computerized tomography (CT) is not possible.

DEVELOPMENT OF ENDOCAVITARY SONOGRAPHY

The desire to close this diagnostic gap led to early attempts to introduce ultrasonic probes working with high frequencies into the body in the hope of obtaining a detailed picture of the gastrointestinal wall and of adjacent tissues. In 1967 the human prostate was demonstrated by the transrectal route using an ultrasonic probe attached on the tip of a rigid rectoscope[1]. The development of endoscopic ultrasound

tomography of the upper gastrointestinal tract was initially characterized by attempts to introduce tiny ultrasonic probes through the
biopsy channel of a flexible gastroscope and by placing then the tip
on the desired position of the gastric mucosa[2]. These probes created
an A-scan that allowed differentiation of large cystic lesions from
solid alterations. However, since the diagnostic value of the one-
dimensional A-scan is very limited this type of endoscopic ultrasonography did not achieve any clinical importance.

For the first time, in 1980, gastroscopes were used with an ultrasonic
probe incorporated in the tip, which generated a B-scan[3,4]. These
probes were either composed of linear ultrasonic elements or they had
a rotating reflector that created a sector scan. Subsequently the sector
scan has achieved major importance in the endosonographic diagnosis
of the upper gastrointestinal (GI) tract, although linear working
devices in combination with forward-viewing endoscopes may also be
used conveniently in selected clinical situations[5].

In the first prototypes the rigid end of the instrument measured
8 cm, and they worked with a frequency of 5 MHz and generated an
85° scan. The latest generation of instruments (Olympus Opt./Aloca;
GFU M2/EUM 2) is characterized by an ultrasonic probe only 2 cm
long with a diameter of 1.3 cm (Fig. 5.1). The device works with a
frequency of 7.5 MHz and generates a 360° endosonographic round-
view (Fig. 5.2) arranged perpendicular to the long axis of the
endoscope. Table 5.1 summarizes the main technical features. At the
present time we are also evaluating scopes that work with a frequency
of 10 MHz.

TECHNIQUE OF INVESTIGATION

The patient is premedicated and examined in the left lateral decubitus
position. The scope is introduced under endoscopic control into the
descending duodenum. The sonographic examination is performed by
slowly pulling back the tip of the instrument, and at the same time
rotating the endoscope around its long axis. The sonographic image is
continuously followed on a monitor. The prerequisite for a satisfactory
image is the undisturbed transmission of the ultrasonic beams. This
may be achieved in two ways. On the one hand a rubber balloon may
be mounted around the sonographic probe, containing about 10 ml of

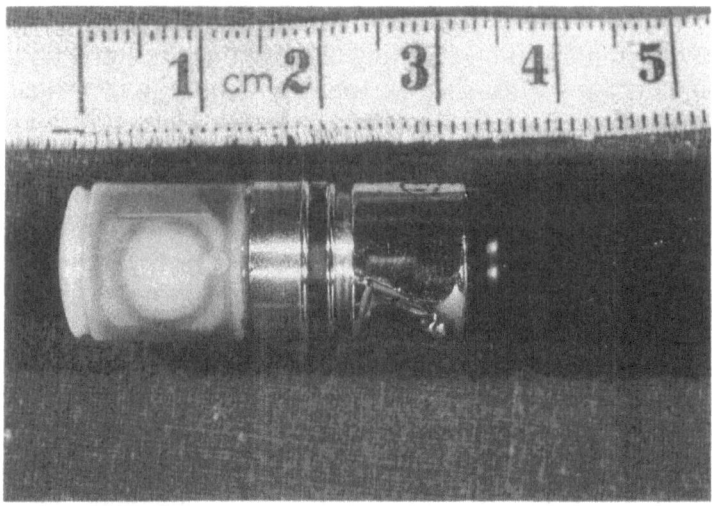

Fig. 5.1 Ultrasonic upper GI endoscope GFU M2/EUM 2 (Olympus Opt./Aloca)

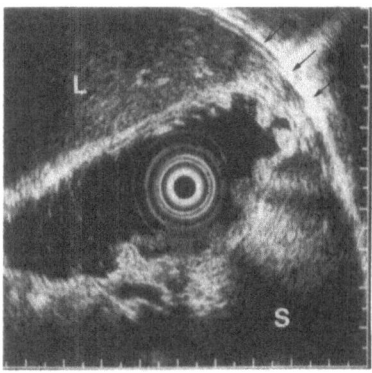

Fig. 5.2 Endosonographic panoramic view from the stomach: L = liver; S = spleen, diaphragm (arrows)

water, thus creating a segment of facilitated ultrasonic beam transmission. This technique is used in the duodenum and prepyloric antrum, as well as in the oesophagus. Investigation of the remaining parts of the stomach is performed after filling this organ with about

Table 5.1 Technical features of the ultrasound endoscope GFU M2/EUM 2 (Olympus/Aloca)

Ultrasound frequency (MHz)	7.5
Rotations (per second)	10
Sector scan (°)	360
Length of rigid end (cm)	4.2
Length of ultrasonic probe (cm)	2
Diameter (cm)	1.3

200 to 300 ml of deaerated water. The probe should be moved to a distance of about 1–2 cm from the gastric wall to keep it in focus. In the stomach this water immersion technique can be combined with the balloon method (Fig. 5.3).

In addition to movements of the endoscope the patient may be placed into different positions to achieve good demonstration of the region of interest. Endosonography of the upper GI tract is a dynamic investigation, and the tip of the instrument is in constant movement due to the peristaltic waves of the stomach and duodenum, the patient's respiratory movements and referred pulsations of the large vessels. Rotation of the tip of the instrument leads to an inversion of the image. These factors make orientation and evaluation of the image difficult. Therefore this technique should be used only by a physician who is well trained in endoscopy and conventional sonography. The duration of the endosonographic investigation should not exceed 30 minutes.

We will first describe the normal findings, and then concentrate on typical endosonographic patterns of pathological lesions in the upper GI tract. Thereafter we will examine the efficacy of this method in selected disorders, and based on these data we will try to elaborate the indications for intraluminal ultrasound of the upper GI tract.

OESOPHAGUS

Due to its tubular form the oesophagus is well suited for endosonographic examination. The evaluation of its wall and the adjacent structures is quite easily accomplished without problems of orientation[6]. The normal oesophageal wall measures about 4–5 mm and displays a typical three-layer pattern. The middle relatively broad

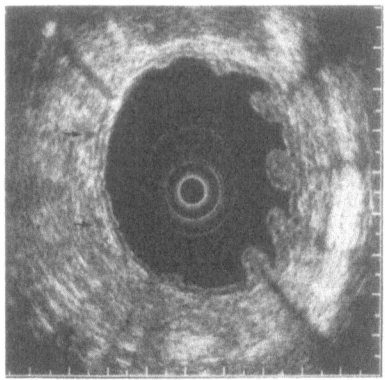

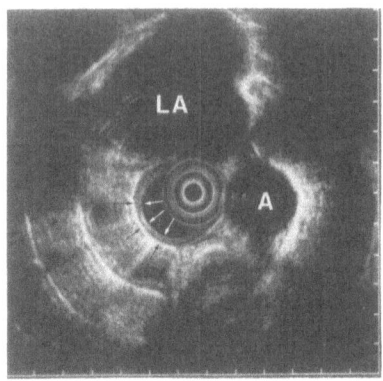

Fig. 5.3 Combined investigation technique in the stomach. Normal gastric wall shown. Note shadows behind gastric folds. Paragastric veins (arrows).

Fig. 5.4 Normal oesophageal wall (between arrows): A = aorta; LA = left atrium

echo-poor layer is believed to correspond to the T. muscularis propria, and is lined by two narrow echogenic bands (Fig. 5.4).

The exact evaluation of the integrity of this echo-poor layer is of great importance for the preoperative staging of oesophageal carcinoma into the prognostically different tumour stages pT2 or pT3. In order to delineate even small alterations of the oesophageal wall the balloon method has to be employed in the examination of the gullet. By doing so compression of intraluminal lesions, e.g. oesophageal varices, is quite frequent, and these dilated vessels may therefore escape endosonographic imaging. However, the demonstration of intramural varices is not affected by inflating the balloon (Fig. 5.5). Oesophageal carcinomas lead to a loss of the normal layer pattern, and to a localized or diffuse thickening of the wall. If tumour stenosis can be passed with the scope the longitudinal extension can be judged, and the transmural view also allows determination of the extension in depth. The penetration of the tumour into the pericardium or into the aorta may be shown or excluded by endosonography (Fig. 5.6). Paraoesophageal echo-poor, round or oval lesions correspond to enlarged lymph nodes and may serve as further evidence of the malignant genesis of the oesophageal lesion. However, in our opinion the sonographic echo pattern does not allow differentiation between

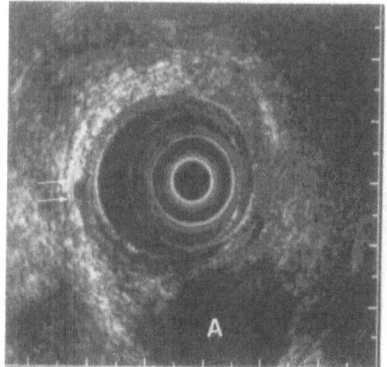 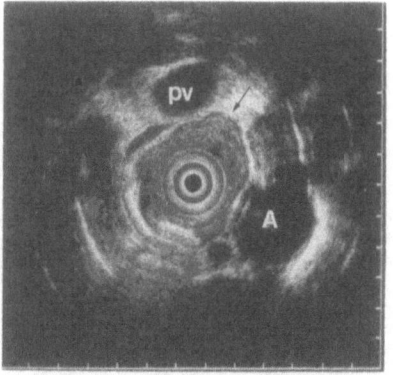

Fig. 5.5 Cross-sectioned oesophageal intramural varicose vein (arrows). On endoscopic examination oesophageal varices °II were seen, that are compressed by the water-filled balloon on endosonographic investigation: A = aorta

Fig. 5.6 Oesophageal carcinoma. Diffuse thickening of the oesophageal wall with an irregular echo pattern. The outer limits are undulated but sharp (arrow): pv = pulmonary vein; A = aorta

benign hyperplastic and metastatically enlarged lymph nodes. Apart from the evaluation of the oesophageal pathology proper, the trans-oesophageal view offers an excellent sonographic window for the demonstration of the adjacent structures. Part of the mediastinum may be evaluated, and alterations of the left atrium, atrial septum, the mitral valve and of the pulmonary veins may be shown[7].

STOMACH

The wall of the stomach may be demonstrated in all parts of the organ, but the corpus is especially well suited. The wall thickness is about 4–6 mm. Endosonographically a five-layer pattern may be discriminated. The inner layer is composed of an inner echogenic and an outer echo-poor band. These sonographic layers are caused by impedance changes from the water-filled lumen to the mucosa with its mucous cover. The middle echogenic layer is probably generated by submucosal structures, whereas the muscular coat of the stomach and the serosa present as an echo-poor and a slim outer echogenic band respectively. The latter is not regularly depicted. If the ultrasonic beam hits a gastric

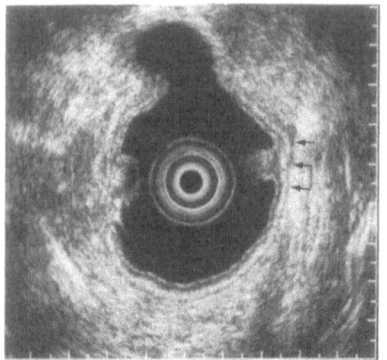 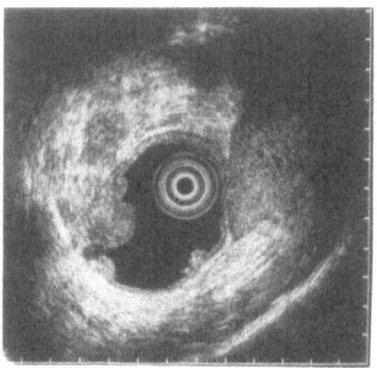

Fig. 5.7 Two polypoid lesions in the stomach. The normal gastric layers are destroyed but the polyp on the right (arrows) does not progress beyond the outer gastric margin, whereas the polyp on the left has destroyed the gastric wall completely and protrudes far into the perigastric tissues and thus fulfils the endosonographic criteria of malignancy.

Fig. 5.8 Polypoid gastric carcinoma. Note echo-poor, irregularly lined paragastric areas, which correspond to metastatic lymph nodes

fold perpendicularly it is scattered, and this leads to a shadow behind the fold with a corresponding extinction of dorsal structures (Fig. 5.3).

Knowing this normal sonographic structure of the stomach polypoid tumours, intramural alterations as well as space-occupying lesions pressing from outside on the gastric wall may be discriminated endosonographically.

Benign lesions are sharply demarcated and do not grow beyond the outer gastric layers. The infiltrative growth of malignant processes leads to a destruction of the gastric wall. The typical layering is no longer discernible, the tumour is irregularly lined (Fig. 5.7). In these cases localized paragastric echo-poor areas correspond to metastatic lymph nodes (Fig. 5.8). In the differential diagnosis of these echo-poor lesions dilated gastric veins caused by portal hypertension must be considered. They are usually smaller than lymph nodes and show a typical 'lined-up' appearance (Fig. 5.9). Prominent gastric folds that do not flatten after introduction of air or water, and give the endoscopic

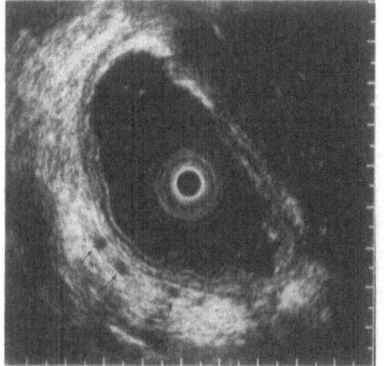 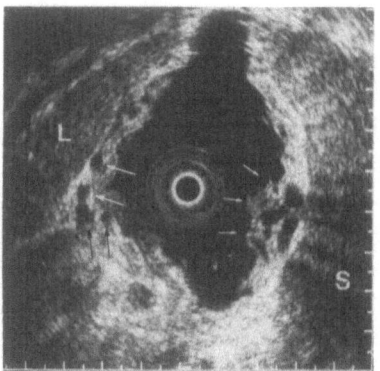

Fig. 5.9 Cross-section of dilated paragastric veins (arrows) in portal hypertension

Fig. 5.10 Prominent gastric fold caused by intramural varicose veins (arrows). Between the liver (L) and the stomach wall several cross-sectioned dilated veins are demonstrated (arrows); S = spleen

impression of being caused by malignant infiltration, e.g. by lymphoma, are quite often caused by dilated varicose veins. By permitting a view of the 'core' of such a lesion these findings are rapidly clarified endosonographically, and a potentially deleterious snare biopsy is avoided (Fig. 5.10). Contractions of the gastric wall and oblique scanning may give the false impression of a thickening of the stomach, and may lead the investigator to the wrong diagnosis of a gastric tumour. Such misinterpretations can be avoided by sufficiently distending the stomach with water and by a meticulous interpretation of all sonographic layers.

PANCREAS

The close contact of the pancreas to the stomach and duodenum makes this organ readily accessible to endosonographic examination. The head of the pancreas is best viewed from the duodenum and from the gastric antrum, while the body and tail regions are delineated by slowly pulling back and straightening the instrument in the gastric corpus (Figs. 5.11 and 5.12). The normal pancreas has a regular echo pattern. Even small (<0.5 cm) pseudocysts may be well delineated

(Fig. 5.13). Calcification of the pancreatic parenchyma and intraductal stones are displayed as bright shadowing echoes. The main pancreatic duct may be evaluated in all its segments and even irregularities of its outer margins as well as dilated small branches are shown by endosonography (Fig. 5.14). Nevertheless, it is difficult to differentiate chronic inflammatory from malignant alterations and the delineation of a malignant tumour in a chronically inflamed organ may even become impossible. Pancreatic carcinomas are usually echo-poor and their local growth, as well as metastatic regional peripancreatic and peribiliary lymph nodes, may be evaluated endosonographically (Fig. 5.15)[8].

GALL BLADDER, BILE DUCTS AND LIVER

The main bile duct may be sharply depicted from the descending duodenum. The dilatation, and often the cause of the obstruction, may be demonstrated. The wall of the common bile duct is composed of three sonographic layers. Stones in the main common bile duct appear as sharp, bright shadowing echoes. The demonstration of space-occupying lesions in the hilum of the liver, as well as of the Klatskin tumour, a carcinoma growing along the bile ducts, are difficult. The gall bladder may be viewed best from the upper portion of the descending duodenum. Even small, tightly packed stones do not produce large irregular echoes, but may be clearly distinguished as individual stones. This sharpness of the picture and the location of the ultrasonic probe close to the gall bladder give rise to the expectation that even tiny polyps of the gall bladder, as well as the infiltrative growth of tumours, will be displayed better, and hopefully earlier, with this method than with conventional techniques[9].

The parts of the liver near to the ultrasonic transducer are depicted well. This holds especially for the left lobe of the liver and adjacent parts of the right lobe. The predetermined and relatively fixed position of the scope inside the duodenum and the gastric antrum, as well as the low tissue penetration of ultrasonic high-frequency beams, are the main reasons that not all parts of the liver can be evaluated.

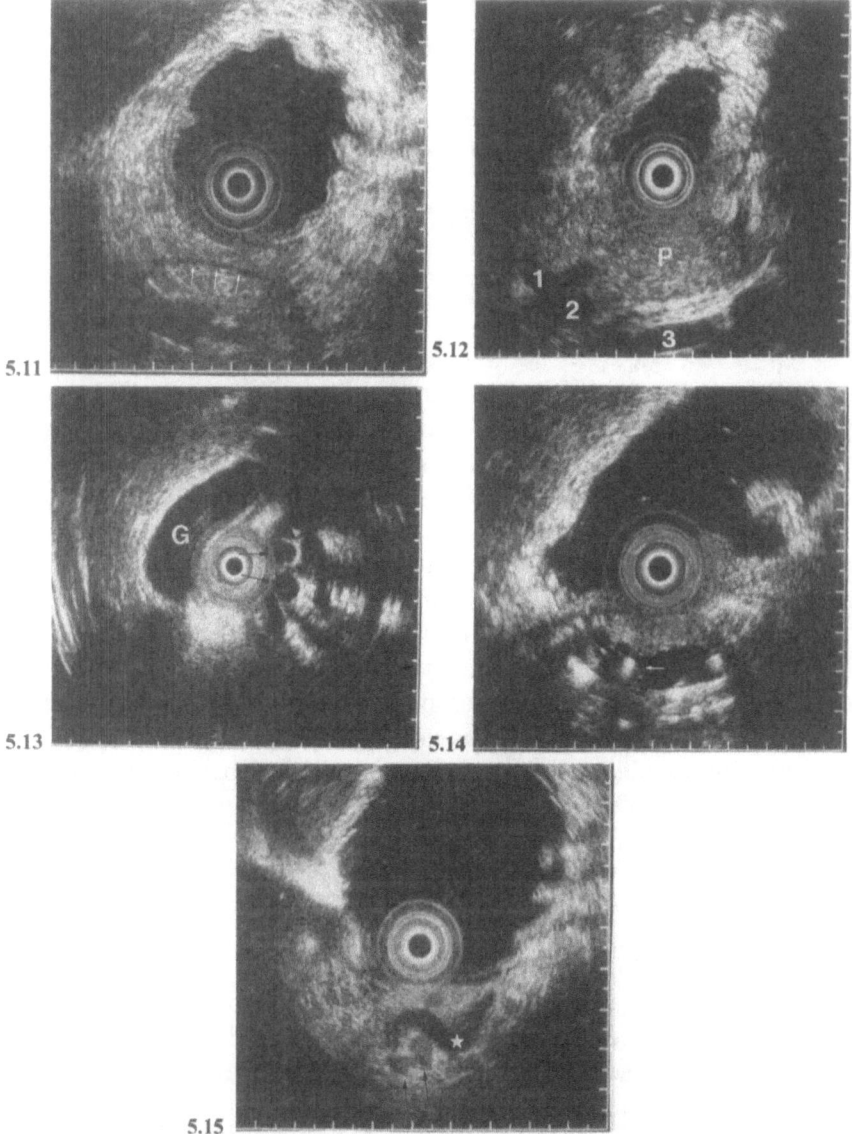

Fig. 5.11 Pancreatic body with normal main pancreatic duct (arrows)
Fig. 5.12 Tail of the pancreas (P): 1 = splenic artery; 2 = splenic vein; 3 = left renal vein
Fig. 5.13 Small pancreatic pseudocysts (arrows): G = gall bladder
Fig. 5.14 Dilated main pancreatic duct. Note the irregularities of its wall. Arrow = intraductal stone
Fig. 5.15 Metastatic lymph nodes (arrows) around coeliac trunk (asterisk)

Table 5.2   Endoscopic sonography in oesophageal diseases ($n = 32$)

Carcinoma	19 (complete passage possible in 7)
Lymphoma	1
Achalasia	6
Submucous tumour	2
Barrett's oesophagus	4

COMPLICATIONS

Complications of endosonographic examinations of the upper GI tract have not been reported, and we did not experience any. Nevertheless sedation of the patient, especially in older persons with chronic obstructive lung disease and cardiocirculatory disorders, can lead to side-effects such as cardiac arrhythmias, a fall in blood pressure and even to respiratory arrest. The necessity to fill the stomach with water carries the risk of an aspiration pneumonia. To diminish this risk we do not perform pharyngeal anaesthesia. Since sonographic scopes are still more rigid than conventional gastroscopes, and are equipped with a side-viewing optic, one must be very careful, especially in the oesophagus, to avoid mucosal lesions or even perforations of fragile carcinomatous tissue. In these cases a radiological barium swallow examination prior to endosonography is recommended, to detect the location and extent of a stricture.

EFFICIENCY OF, AND INDICATIONS FOR, ENDOSCOPIC ULTRASOUND

Before a new method can be introduced into clinical practice its value has to be compared to already existing methods, and its efficacy has to be shown in defined clinical settings. Many publications regarding endoscopic ultrasound deal with the diagnostic potential of this method. It should therefore be welcome that, especially in the recent past, controlled studies have been performed to evaluate the diagnostic efficiency of this technique.

The diagnosis of *oesophageal carcinoma* has been made correctly by Heyder et al.[9] in 27 out of 30 cases. We have performed endo-sonography studies on 32 patients with diseases of the oesophagus (Table 5.2)[10]. Nineteen patients had histologically proven carcinoma of the oesophagus and the diagnosis was known beforehand to the investigator. Endosonography was performed to assess the preoperative staging capability of the method. Based on the sonographic criteria mentioned above, the carcinoma could be demonstrated endosonographically in all cases. However, passage of tumour stricture was possible only in seven of the 19 cases. Benign submucous tumours could be seen in two cases, and in six patients with stenosis due to achalasia a tumour was excluded endosonographically after pneumodilatation in five patients. Four patients with Barrett's oesophagus are regularly followed up by endosonography. Although in one case cytological brushings led to the suspicion of a malignant tumour, on endosonography the entire wall of the oesophagus was smooth. The patient was not operated on, and the clinical course in this case confirmed the endosonographic diagnosis. In a second case cytologically dysplastic cells were described. On endosonography a localized thickening of the oesophageal wall was demonstrated, and was confirmed at operation to be a carcinoma. In the follow-up of patients with an endobrachyoesophagus endosonography represents a valuable additional tool.

Although in cases of known oesophageal carcinoma the nature of the stenosis was assessed correctly, preoperative staging of the carcinoma by endosonography at the present time is limited, since tumour stricture cannot be passed in the majority of cases, and thus it is impossible to evaluate tumour tissue beyond the stenosis. These results, however, should not be discouraging, since they are only partly due to the method itself. They rather mirror the clinical problem that, in most patients seen by us, the oesophageal carcinoma was already far progressed. Controlled studies by Japanese authors[11] demonstrate that endosonography at the present time is the most sensitive tool in the delineation of the extension of small oesophageal tumours. When early diagnosis is made, excellent long-term results will be obtained. It is well known that oesophageal cancer spreads both longitudinally and circumferentially in the oesophageal wall. Submucosal spread is beyond endoscopic visibility, and although CT and magnetic resonance imaging have made staging before operation more accurate, demonstration of submucosal spread often is missed by these methods. The logical consequence of our results therefore seems to be to apply endosonography early in the diagnostic evaluation of dysphagia. In our hospital each dysphagia whose aetiology is not clarified completely by endoscopy, radiology or neurological examination represents an indication for endosonographic evaluation.

The possibility of determining the depth of infiltration of *gastric tumours* justifies the hope that endosonography will also play an important role in this clinical setting[12]. First reports dealing with the diagnostic value of endosonography in early gastric cancer are promising. Takemoto's group even treats the endosonographically verified early carcinoma without metastases with endoscopic laser. At the present time, however, a final judgement in this regard is not possible.

The demonstration of extragastric lesions that impress the gastric wall will also be a domain of endosonography, although large controlled studies regarding this issue are not available. The delineation of the pancreatic body and tail succeeds regularly. Since, however, with the presently available instruments the pyloric passage is only possible in about 80% of cases a systematic approach to the head of the pancreas and to the papilla Vateri is not possible regularly. Our investigations[13] of the efficiency of endosonographic diagnosis of *benign pancreatic and biliary lesions* demonstrate that of 87 examined patients 12 had a chronic calcifying pancreatitis, eight of whom also had pseudocysts. In all 12 cases the diagnosis could be made correctly with endosonography, and in addition it was possible to demonstrate even small pseudocysts, diameter was less than 0.5 cm, which were not seen by CT or sonography. Even small exudates in the omental bursa not visualized by other methods were visible endosonographically. The clinical importance of such a finding remains to be defined. Eighteen of our patients had a dilated common bile duct that could be seen, at least partially, endosonographically, and in seven out of eight cases stones in the main bile duct were demonstrated endosonographically. A histologically proven adenomyosis of Vater's papilla escaped endosonographic demonstration in three patients. We examined three cases with the clinical manifestations of *hormone-producing pancreatic tumours*. An insulinoma, 1.5 cm in diameter, and a large glucagonoma in the pancreatic tail were seen by endosonography. These tumours were also demonstrable with conventional methods. A small insulinoma (0.5 cm diameter) in the dorsal part of the pancreatic head could not be seen on endosonography or with conventional ultrasound, computed tomography, angiography or nuclear magnetic resonance. The tumour was finally localized during operation by the palpating finger of the surgeon. The experiences of other investigators[14] show, however, that thanks to the excellent detailed resolution of endosonography even small APUDomas are demonstrable. Yet the total number of cases reported in the literature is too small to permit a final judgement at the present time.

In 118 patients examined by endosonography Yasuda *et al.*[15] found a *pancreatic carcinoma* in 13 cases. Nine of these tumours were larger than 3 cm in diameter, one had a diameter of 2.5 cm, and in the remaining three cases the tumour was smaller than 2 cm. All these tumours were echo-poor. In 10 of these 13 cases, besides conventional and endoscopic ultrasound ERCP, computed tomography and angiography were also performed. The positive finding rate of endosonography reported by the authors was 100%, for conventional ultrasound 40%, for ERCP 80%, computed tomography 70% and for angiography 80%. None of the three tumours smaller than 2 cm showed any metastases and could be resected curatively. From these studies the authors conclude that, compared to ERCP, CT, angiography and conventional ultrasound, 'endosonography is the most useful method for the demonstration of small pancreatic carcinomas of less than 20 mm size'. In a further prospective study[16] aimed at investigating the sensitivity and specificity of endosonography compared to conventional morphological methods in the diagnosis of pancreatic cancer, 34 patients with painless jaundice were examined. Endosonography was performed after conventional ultrasound. Three tumours of Vater's papilla were detected by endosonography, and conventional ultrasound demonstrated only one of them. Ten pancreatic cancers with a mean size of 2.8 cm were diagnosed by endosonography. According to the authors endosonography permitted a more precise description of outer tumour margins and of its inner echo structure compared to conventional ultrasound, so that in addition to the demonstration of a pathological lesion endosonographic criteria allowed better discrimination between benign and malignant alterations. Six of their cases were echo-poor, two echo-dense and two showed a mixed reflex pattern. It was remarkable that four malignant tumours showed smooth outer contours. Both studies cited are laudable efforts to assess objectively the diagnostic efficiency of endosonography in the diagnosis of pancreatic cancer. The endosonographic demonstration of a large tumour that has already been visualized by other methods is, of course, of no prognostic advantage to the patient. An interesting starting point for further prospective studies that must aim at the endosonographic diagnosis of potentially curatively resectable tumours is the ability of the method to demonstrate small tumours that escape delineation with conventional methods[17]. However, due to the natural course of pancreatic carcinoma a systematic early detection of this neoplasia with endoscopic ultrasound is not to be expected. In this case, too, endosonography is to be viewed as a complementary method.

The excellent capability of conventional ultrasound in the diagnosis of *cholecystolithiasis* makes an endosonographic examination in these cases superfluous. Since, however, the gall bladder is frequently visualized during examinations performed for other reasons the high detail resolution of this method will again be evident. The same is true for the *liver*, that is clearly seen with conventional ultrasound, and therefore it is not to be expected that endosonography will play an important role in the diagnosis of liver diseases. Nevertheless it is worthwhile to perform endosonographic study of tumours of the bile ducts that are localized in the hilum of the liver, or spread in the hepatoduodenal ligament and infiltrate the porta hepatis. Clinical experience shows that these tumours are not visualized by sonography, computed tomography, angiography or nuclear magnetic resonance, although they might have already attained a large size. Stenosis, and proximal dilatation of the bile ducts, are frequently the only indirect tumour signs, and a short stenosis is often caused by a tumour that proves to be irresectable. It would mean tangible progress if it became possible, with endosonography, to delineate tumour size accurately before operation.

CONCLUSIONS AND A LOOK TO THE FUTURE

From the preceding sections it should have become clear that endoscopic sonography of upper GI tract in most clinical settings is still to be regarded as a clinical experimental method. The indications for an endosonographic examination should be restricted (Table 5.3). They must be deduced from the technical features of the method, namely

Table 5.3   Indications for endoscopic sonography of the upper GI tract

Oesophagus	Dysphagia
	Barrett's oesophagus
	Achalasia (after dilatation)
	Submucous tumours
	Carcinoma
Stomach	Intraluminal and submucous tumours
	Extragastric impressions
	Carcinoma
	Lymphoma
	Ménétrier's gastritis
	'Prominent folds' of unknown etiology
Pancreas	Search for small (<2 cm) carcinoma
	Tumours of Vater's papilla
	Hormone-producing tumours

high detail resolution and low penetration of the ultrasonic beam. We expect that endosonography will be helpful in planning palliative laser treatment and radiation-afterloading therapy of oesophageal cancers by accurately describing the depth of tumour invasion. Additional information will also be gained from endosonography in portal hypertension. Thus potentially deleterious snare biopsies of prominent folds seen on gastroscopy will be avoided by a prior endosonographic examination that shows such folds to be made up of intramural varicose vessels.

The procedure is not to be regarded as an alternative to conventional ultrasound, and endosonography should only be performed to assess the wall of the GI tract itself, or tissues and organs in its immediate proximity. Since the procedure requires a fair amount of endoscopic and sonographic skill the method should only be performed by physicians well trained in these techniques. Complications have not been reported yet, but due to the premedication should be kept in mind, especially in older patients with cardiac and pulmonary diseases. Filling the stomach with water carries the risk of an aspiration pneumonia.

Unquestionably marked technical progress has been achieved in recent years, and technical developments will lead to further noticeable improvements in endoscopic ultrasound. The aim must be to reduce the diameter of the scopes, to make the instruments more flexible and, in addition to side-viewing instruments, forward-viewing endoscopes equipped with ultrasonic probes should be introduced. The latter should provide a sector scan image even if this leads to a modest reduction of the 360° view. The presently available mechanical scanners should be replaced by electronic devices. We assume that in future the effort to perform an endosonographic examination will be comparable to a 'simple' gastroscopy with the opportunity to obtain tissue biopsies, to perform transmural fine-needle biopsies and to switch on the endosonographic transducer as required. These major breakthroughs will lead to an increase in the use of endosonography in clinical routine.

References

1. Watanabe, H., Kato, H., Kato, T., Tanaka, M. and Teresawa, Y. (1986). Diagnostic application of the ultrasonography for the prostate. *Jpn. J. Urol.*, **59**, 273
2. Lutz, H and Rösch, W. (1976). Transgastroscopic ultrasonography. *Endoscopy*, **8**, 203–5
3. Di Magno, E. P., Buxton, J. L., Regan, P. T., Hattery, R. R., Wilson, D. A., Suarez, J. R. and Green, R. S. (1980). The ultrasonic endoscope. *Lancet*, **1**, 629–31
4. Di Magno, E. P., Regan, P. T., Clain, J. E., James, E. M. and Buxton, J. L. (1982). Human endoscopic ultrasonography. *Gastroenterology*, **83**, 824–9
5. Lilienfeld-Toal, H. V. and Kampmann, B. (1985). Endoskopische Ultraschalluntersuchung des Oesophagus. *Dtsch. Med. Wochenschr.*, **110**, 1554
6. Strohm, W. D. and Classen, M. (1985). Endoskopische Ultraschalluntersuchung des Oesophagus. *Dtsch. Med. Wochenschr.*, **110**, 783–8
7. Reifart, N. W., Strohm, D. and Classen, M. (1983). Die endoskopische Echokardiographie. *Herz u. Gefässe*, **3**, 688–94
8. Tio, T. L. and Tytgat, G. N. (1984). Endoscopic ultrasonography in the assessment of intra- and trans-mural infiltration of tumors in the esophagus, stomach and papilla of Vater and in the detection of extra-esophageal lesions. *Endoscopy*, **16**, 203–10
9. Heyder, N., Lux, G., Riemann, J. F. and Lutz, H. (1986). Ultraschall-Endoskopie. Eine Bestandsaufnahme nach 3 Jahren. *Dtsch. Med. Wochenschr.*, **111**, 324–8

10. Dancygier, H. and Classen, M. (1986). How can we diagnose the depth of cancer invasion in the esophagus? *Endoscopy,* **18** (Suppl. 3), 19–21
11. Takemoto, T., Ito, T., Aibe, T. and Okita, K. (1986). Endoscopic ultrasonography in the diagnosis of esophageal carcinoma with particular regard to staging it for operability. *Endoscopy,* **18** (Suppl. 3), 22–5
12. Caletti, G., Bolondi, L., Brocchi, E., Casanova, P., Zani, L., Gaiani, S., Testa, S., Guizzardi, G. and Labo, G. (1983). Staging of gastric cancer by means of endoscopic ultrasonography. *Gut,* **24,** A493–4
13. Dancygier, H. and Classen, M. (1986). Endosonographic diagnosis of benign pancreatic and biliary lesions. *Scand. J. Gastroenterol.,* **21** (Suppl. 123), 119–22
14. Heyder, N. (1985). Localization of an insulinoma by ultrasonic endoscopy *N. Engl. J. Med.,* **312,** 860
15. Yasuda, K., Tanaka, Y., Fujimoto, S., Nakajima, M. and Kawai, K. (1984). Use of endoscopic ultrasonography in small pancreatic cancer. *Scand. J. Gastroenterol.,* **19** (Suppl. 102), 9
16. Strohm, W. D., Kurtz, W., Hagenmüller, F. and Classen, M. (1984). Diagnostic efficacy of endoscopic ultrasound tomography in pancreatic cancer and cholestasis. *Scand. J. Gastroenterol.,* **19** (Suppl. 102), 18–23
17. Dancygier, H. and Classen, M. (1986). Endoscopic sonography of pancreatic cancer. *Front. Gastrointest. Res.,* **12,** 195–207
18. Dancygier, H. and Classen, M. (1986). Endoskopische Sonographie des oberen Verdauungstraktes. *Med. Klinik,* **81,** 92–6
19. Dancygier, H. and Classen, M. (1986). Endoskopische Sonographie – ein diagnostischer Fortschritt im oberen Verdauungstrakt? *Leber Magen Darm.,* **16,** 114–20

Index